ECHINACEA

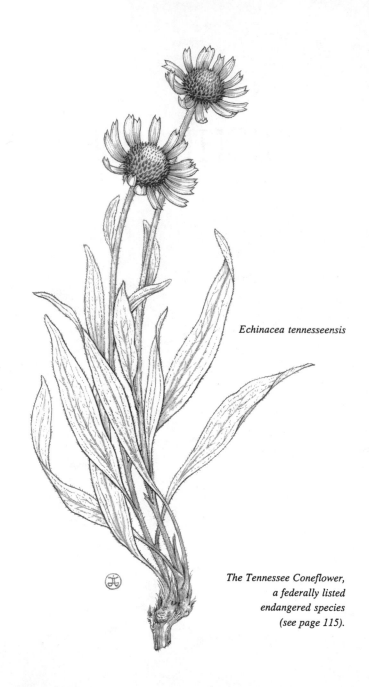

Echinacea tennesseensis

*The Tennessee Coneflower,
a federally listed
endangered species
(see page 115).*

ECHINACEA
Nature's Immune Enhancer

Steven Foster

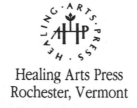

Healing Arts Press
Rochester, Vermont

Healing Arts Press
One Park Street
Rochester, Vermont 05767

Originally published as *Echinacea Exalted: The Botany, Culture, History and Medicinal Uses of the Purple Coneflower* by the Ozark Beneficial Plant Project, Ozark Resource Center, Brixey, Missouri. First edition 1984. Second edition 1985.

Library of Congress Cataloging-in-Publication Data
Foster, Steven, 1957-
   Echinacea : nature's immune enhancer / Steven Foster ; illustrated by Judith Ann Griffith.
      p.   cm.
   Rev. ed. of: Echinacea exalted. 2nd ed., rev. and enl. Brixey, Mo.
: Ozark Beneficial Plant Project, Ozark Resource Center, c1985.
   Includes bibliographical references.
   ISBN 0-89281-386-5 (paper)
   1. Echinacea (Plants) --Therapeutic use. 2. Echinacea (Plants)
I. Foster, Steven, 1957- Echinacea exalted. II. Title.
RS165.E4F67 1990
615'.32355--dc20   90-24824
                                                      CIP

Printed and bound in the United States

10 9 8 7 6 5 4

Healing Arts Press is a division of Inner Traditions International, Ltd.

Distributed to the book trade in the United States by American International Distribution Corporation (AIDC)

Distributed to the book trade in Canada by Book Center, Inc., Montreal, Quebec

Distributed to the health food trade in Canada by Alive Books, Toronto and Vancouver

Cover illustration: Line drawing of *Echinacea paradoxa* var. *neglecta*

*Dedicated to the conservation of
indigenous populations of Echinacea*

A portion of the author's proceeds from the sale of this
work goes to support Echinacea conservation and
research projects of the Ozark Beneficial
Plant Project Ozarks Resource Center
Brixey, MO 65618

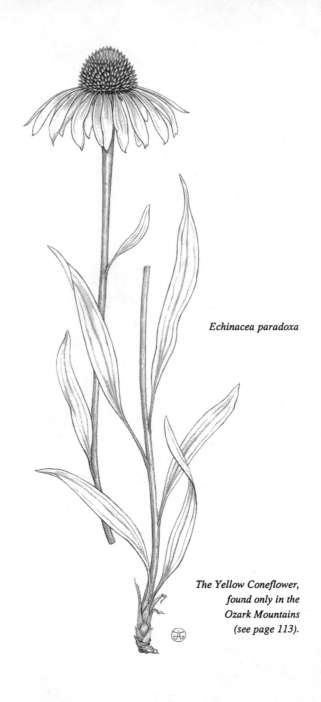

Echinacea paradoxa

*The Yellow Coneflower,
found only in the
Ozark Mountains
(see page 113).*

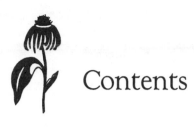

Contents

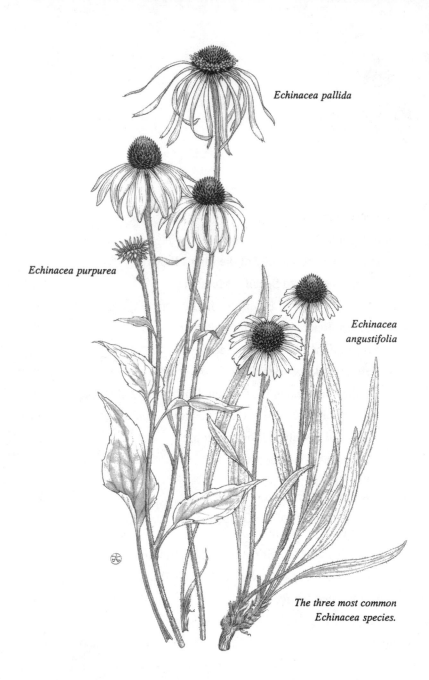

Echinacea pallida

Echinacea purpurea

*Echinacea
angustifolia*

The three most common
Echinacea species.

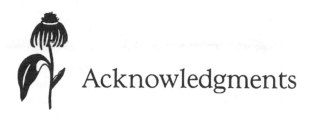

Acknowledgments

The two previous editions of this publication were produced under the auspices of the Ozark Beneficial Plant Project, Ozarks Resource Center, Brixey, Missouri, aided in part by grants from the Threshold Foundation. The former title was *Echinacea Exalted—The Botany, Culture, History and Medicinal Uses of the Purple Coneflowers*.

The following individuals have contributed information or inspiration to the work in one form or another: Mark Blumenthal, American Botanical Council; Connie Cloak, Cheekwood Botanical Gardens; Ed Croom, Research Institute of Pharmaceutical Science, The University of Mississippi; Dr. James A. Duke, ARS, USDA; Henry Gilbert, National Agricultural Library, USDA; Dr. Marshall Johnston, University of Texas, Austin; Dr. Paul Lee; Steve Moring, Botanica Analytica; Dr. Gerald A. Myers, South Dakota State University; Ruth B. Quimby, NAPRALERT, University of Illinois at Chicago; Ed Smith, Herb-Pharm; Dr. Paul Somers, Tennessee Natural Heritage Division, Department of Conservation; Dr. Connie Taylor, Southeastern Oklahoma State University; Ginnie Wallace and Dr. James H. Wilson, Missouri Department of Conservation; Connie Wolf, Library, Missouri Botanical Garden.

The author would like to express his deep gratitude to the following individuals who have supplied valuable help. Dr. Habil. Rudolf Bauer, Institute for Pharmaceutical Biology, University of Munich, the leading researcher on pharmaceutical aspects of Echinacea, generously fulfilled any request I presented for references and commentaries. Dr. Brent Davis, Wildwood Botanics, sparked my initial Echinacea interest-turned-passion. Dr. William J. Dress, L. H. Bailey Hortorium, Cornell University, supplied valuable information on cultivation. Thomas Hemmerly, Middle Tennessee State University, supplied useful information on the Tennessee Coneflower. Christopher Hobbs, Institute for Natural Products Research, who has unlocked the obscure and foreign-language literature on Echinacea for an American audience, freely provided research materials and feedback. Lon Johnson, Trout Lake Farm, shared his experience as a grower and marketer. Kelly Kindscher, University of Kansas, shared notes and references on ethnobotanical aspects. Dr. Ronald L. McGregor, University of Kansas, was quick to provide references, knowledge, germplasm, and the general wisdom of his vast experience in the botany of Echinacea. Rebecca Perry, Lloyd Library and Museum, provided numerous hard-to-find references and library service efficient beyond expectations. Dr. R. Liersch and Dr. W. Krümke, Madaus AG, provided information on dozens of German Echinacea studies.

Judith Ann Griffith is gratefully acknowledged for supplying her exquisite pen and inks to illustrate this work.

Sasha Daucus is deeply appreciated for her translations of numerous German articles.

Special thanks to Anne Bartley, Alan Slifka, Nancy Ward, Denise Henderson, Ceil Lilyquist, Vinnie McKinney, Louise Wienckowski, and the Ozark Beneficial Plant Project of the Ozarks Resource Center, whose support made this publication possible.

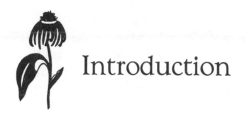

Introduction

This [herb], which has slowly wedged its way into attention, is persistently forcing itself into conspicuity. The probabilities are that in a time to come, it will be ardently sought and widely used, for it is not one of the multitude that have flashed into sight, been artfully pushed, then investigated, found wanting, and next dropped out of sight and out of mind.

J. U. Lloyd (1904a, p. 9)

Those words, written over eighty years ago by John Uri Lloyd, the most important writer in the history of North American medical botany, have proven true.

It may be difficult to imagine common threads between the cultures of the Indians who once freely roamed the Midwest prairies and the high-tech culture of modern West Germany. One of the most important medicinal plants of the Indian groups of the Plains is today one of the most widely used herbal products in West Germany. Over the past fifty years, scientists, primarily in Germany, have investigated and in many cases confirmed a rational scientific basis for the traditional medicinal uses of this plant group. That research has catapulted it from the status of a snakebite remedy to classification as a nonspecific stimulant to the immune defense system. This plant group is the genus Echinacea (pronounced ek-i-NAY-see-a), or the Purple Coneflowers. The name is derived from the Greek word root *echinos,* meaning hedgehog or sea urchin (the evolution of the genus' botanical names is discussed in chapter 11).

1

Echinacea, a genus of the aster family (Compositae or Asteraceae), is represented by nine species found only in the United States and south central Canada. They occur from Massachusetts to Georgia and west to Texas and eastern Montana. Six of the nine species have relatively narrow natural ranges. Two species are very rare, including the federally listed endangered species, the Tennessee Coneflower *Echinacea tennesseensis,* known from only five populations. A rare Appalachian species, *Echinacea laevigata,* is under review for endangered species status. The Yellow Coneflower *Echinacea paradoxa* and the purple-flowered *Echinacea simulata* are found only in the Ozarks of Arkansas and Missouri. *Echinacea sanguinea* occurs in the West Gulf Coast Plain of Louisiana and eastern Texas. *Echinacea atrorubens* has a very narrow range in extreme eastern Kansas and Oklahoma.

The three most widely distributed species have a long tradition of medicinal use. The Common Purple Coneflower *Echinacea purpurea* grows sporadically throughout much of eastern North America and is widely grown as a garden ornamental. Pale Purple Coneflower *Echinacea pallida* occurs in the Midwest. The Narrow-leaved Purple Coneflower *Echinacea angustifolia* occurs throughout much of the western Great Plains.

As a medicinal plant group, the genus Echinacea has gone through periods of favor and disfavor. It was probably used by the Plains Indians for more purposes than any other plant. Introduced to the medical profession in 1887, from the turn of the century into the 1930s it became the best-selling American medicinal plant among physicians in the United States. The middle decades of this century found the use of Echinacea waning, primarily as the result of the introduction of sulfa drugs and antibiotics such as penicillin, but in the last decade, interest in the plant group has dramatically increased, particularly among health professionals, herbalists, the herb-consuming public, and researchers in botany, horticulture, phytochemistry, and pharmacology. The research conducted over the past fifty years reveals new findings that could catapult it into prominence as a potential treatment for minor and severe infections, viral afflictions, and as a nonspecific stimulant to the immune defense system.

Today this plant, once used for more ailments than any other by American Indians and popularly prescribed by medical practitioners in the early part of this century, has again gained popularity in the United States in the form of a wide variety of products available in health and natural food markets. Its greatest popularity, however, is now in Europe, particularly West Germany, where over 280 Echinacea products and phytopharmaceuticals (plant-based medicines) are made.

Botanical medicine has always been strong in Germany and has lived side by side with better known and more widely accepted Western medical modalities. Despite the fact that forty plant species provide ingredients for 25 percent of all prescription medicines sold in the United States today, there is proportionately very little money spent on medicinal plant research in this country. Many studies on American medicinal plants are now performed by German scientists, with the results published in German scientific periodicals.

Why must we turn to the Germans for information on American medicinal plants? Simply put, in Germany there is a continuous tradition of herbal medicine as well as accepted herb use in Western or allopathic medicine. In the United States, we have a broken tradition of herb use. This schism is the result of social and economic factors, as well as unrealistic federal regulations that hamper research in herbal medicines by rendering such research unprofitable for American pharmaceutical companies.

For any substance to be labeled as a "drug" in the United States, that is, to be allowed to make claims for medicinal use on the label or in promotional literature, the substance must be proven both "safe and effective" before it receives FDA approval. Under these regulations, it costs well over $125 million to bring a single new drug into the American marketplace. This cost, of course, limits research to only the largest of pharmaceutical firms—and only to products that promise a high rate of return on the enormous investment.

A large proportion of pharmaceutical research for new drug development is funded by pharmaceutical companies. For this effort, the government rewards them with exclusive patent rights on a new drug for twenty-two years after it has been proven safe and effective and then approved for sale by the FDA. Therefore, American drug companies are only interested in new drug research if the final outcome can be protected by patents. While a synthetic chemical modeled on plant compounds or a novel method for extracting natural compounds could be patented, basic research on plant drugs does not result in new drug applications. As a result, medicinal plant research is at a virtual standstill in the United States compared to other countries.

In this country, work on medicinal plants has largely focused on the discovery of powerful chemical components such as the heart-regulating glycosides of Foxglove *(Digitalis* spp.); reserpine, a tranquilizing drug derived from Indian Snake Root *(Rauwolfia serpentina);* and the alkaloids of the Madagascar Periwinkle *(Catharanthus roseus),* which are used in the chemotherapy for the treatment of Hodgkin's disease and several forms of childhood leukemia. Developed in the mid 1960s by the Eli Lilly Company, the drugs from the Madagascar Periwinkle were the last major plant-derived drugs developed in the United States. Despite the fact that forty plant species provide ingredients for 25 percent of all prescription medicines sold in the United States today, there is proportionately very little money spent on medicinal plant research in the United States.

According to Norman R. Farnsworth and D. D. Soejarto of the Programme for Collaborative Research in the Pharmaceutical Sciences of the College of Pharmacy, University of Illinois, Chicago, prescription drugs enjoyed over $8 billion in retail consumer sales in 1981, but less than $200,000 was spent by pharmaceutical companies in researching new drugs from plants. Dr. Farnsworth calls his scientific discipline, known as pharmacognosy, an endangered species in North American academia. Pharmacognosy is the scientific discipline dealing with the study of drugs from natural sources (Farnsworth and Soejarto 1985).

In an article in the July–September 1985 issue of *Economic Botany*, "Potential Consequence of Plant Extinction in the United States on the Current and Future Availability of Prescription Drugs," Farnsworth and Soejarto point out that while Japanese scientists investigate Japanese plants, Chinese scientists research Chinese plants, and Soviet researchers study Russian plants, "American scientists, for some strange reason, rarely investigate American plants as a source of drugs" (Farnsworth and Soejarto 1985).

A major reason for the lack of successful development of new plant drugs in the United States in the late twentieth century, stated by Dr. Varro E. Tyler, a prominent pharmacognosist and vice president of Purdue University, is lack of effective cooperation among researchers in applicable biological, physical and clinical sciences. A broad multidisciplinary effort is necessary for the development of new plant drugs. This includes many scientific disciplines, including plant taxonomy, ethnobotany (the study of plant uses among indigenous peoples), pharmacognosy, biochemistry, analytical chemistry, pharmacology, and clinical medicine. Few organizations, including the largest pharmaceutical firms, educational institutions, and government agencies, have the opportunity to bring this large and diverse number of scientific disciplines together to tackle a single problem (Tyler 1986).

Despite current problems, Dr. Tyler also outlines new, simpler methods of assaying biological compounds and the future development of less expensive and more exact analytical equipment as a bright spot for the future. Dr. Tyler and his coauthors state a similar case in their introductory chapter to the ninth edition of the textbook *Pharmacognosy*. Part of the answer, the authors suggest, is government regulations strict enough to protect public health without stifling innovative research (Tyler, Brady, and Robbers 1988). As author of *The New Honest Herbal*, Dr Tyler is well known as one of the most conservative voices in the scientific community on medicinal herb use. While his views on the use of herbs are considered conservative by many herbalists, his approach to the regulation of herbs in the United States is progessive.

In Germany things are different. As Dr. Tyler (1986) notes, the use of natural drugs (or herbs) in Germany has always been a strong tradition and continues to prevail. He quotes a survey showing that 76 percent of German women used herbal teas for healthful benefits. Fifty-two percent of persons surveyed used herbal remedies for the treatment of minor ailments. In addition to the strong and continued tradition of herb use for medicinal purposes the regulatory climate is more favorable. As in the United States, herb products must be proven safe and effective before they are sold to the German public. They are also standardized, containing predictable amounts of properly identified whole plant materials (leaf, root, bark, etc.), or active chemical components. If an herb has been used safely for a long period of time, reasonable certainty of efficacy and safety is substituted for the expensive toxicological, pharmacological, and clinical research required in the United States. Great emphasis is placed on clinical reports of experienced practitioners, supplemented by literature reports, and data supplied by product manufacturers. The regulations in Germany provide financial incentives for relatively small companies to research and innovate in developing new medicinal herb products. These incentives stimulate competition and encourage new product development, supplying safe and effective, properly labeled, standardized products (Tyler 1979). And some, like Echinacea, are American medicinal plants!

Such a positive regulatory situation is not unique to Germany. Rational regulations for medicinal herbal product use exist in several European countries and, as of 1990, in Canada as well. In Canada, herbal product manufacturers can apply for a drug identification number (DIN), a Canadian regulatory category equivalent to the over-the-counter (OTC) category in the United States. If safety and efficacy can be established in literature reviews and other data supplied by the manufacturer, a DIN is awarded, and traditional medicinal claims can be placed on the product label.

On 12 October 1989, by invitation of the Health Protection Branch, Health and Welfare Canada, Dr. Tyler gave a lecture entitled, "The Herbal Regulatory Dilemma: A Proposed Solution." For herbs to become generally accepted for medicinal use in our society certain conditions assuring proper identification, labeling, and quality standards must be met. Basically, Dr. Tyler's position was fourfold: (1) Prepare a "Botanical Codex or similar compendium to establish standards of identity, purity, and quality for all crude vegetable drugs"; (2) Mandate "that all herbs sold be properly identified by their Latin binomial, and that a method of determining compliance with appropriate standards be implemented"; (3) Establish "the safety . . . of all herbs sold to consumers"; (4) Allow "herbs to be sold with approved traditional claims of efficacy, provided all the other requirements have been met."

I believe that Dr. Tyler's fourfold position on regulation is what we need to make higher quality, properly labeled herb products available to a wide cross section of American consumers. While not sold or labeled as "drugs," many herb products, including dozens of Echinacea products, are available in the United States, primarily in health and natural food outlets. Rather than being sold as drugs, they are sold as "foods" or "supplements." Unfortunately, current regulations in the United States, instead of allowing traditional health claims to be made for such products, in effect require them to be mislabeled and thwart the manufacturer from presenting information on the intended use of the product.

Regulations may also prevent proper labeling of the actual product form. Alcohol extracts, or tinctures, have become increasingly available over the past ten years. The FDA frowns upon the use of the term "tincture" in herb product labeling, regarding the use of the term itself as "drug labeling." Some district FDA offices have forced small tincture manufacturers to drop the term "tincture" from herb product labels. Products that are by all definitions (except the FDA's) "tinctures" must instead be labeled "lotion" if for external use, or "drops", "extracts," or other names if to be ingested internally. While the FDA is charged with protecting American consumers, in this case a disservice is forced upon the consumers by requiring that manufacturers call their products something different than what they really are.

In 1986, Dr. Tyler observed that there will probably be a change in the United States regulatory environment as health-conscious consumers gain more accurate information on herbs and demand wider availability of natural products.

The problems of medicinal plant research and development, as well as the stifling regulatory dilemma in the United States, have historical roots based in the climate of nineteenth-century medical practice in America, where various groups of physicians or medical practitioners competed for clients and prominence. The historical introduction, use, development, and the eventual demise of the use of Echinacea from the 1930s to the 1970s are all intricately woven into the fabric of American medical history.

Nineteenth-century medical practitioners included: "allopathic" or regular physicians, the tradition that produced modern Western medicine; homeopathic physicians, followers of the medical system of the eighteenth-century German physician, Samuel Hahnemann; eclectic physicians who, as the name implies, used a combination of medical modalities, but who especially relied on the use of American medicinal plants; and other groups, such as Thomsonian physicians, followers of the medical system developed by the self-taught New Hampshire native, Samuel Thomson.

Reaction against the dramatic therapies employed by allopathic physicians in the late eighteenth and early nineteenth century, such as the copious use of mercury preparations, opium, and blood letting, helped give rise to various groups of "alternative" medical practitioners. Principles of Jacksonian democracy, which included glorification of the common man, individualism, laissez-faire sentiments, fear of monopolies, hatred of corporations, and other complex social and economic factors, helped set the stage for the rise of the Thomsonian physicians, who flourished in the first half of the nineteenth century. The founder of the movement, Samuel Thomson (1769–1843), sold "family rights" to his system of medicine by subscription, for $20 per family. The Thomsonians treated all disease in the same manner. The basic objective was to "balance inward and outward heat." This was accomplished with a "course" of treatments, including the use of steam baths, large doses of Lobelia *(Lobelia inflata)*, heat stimulants such as cayenne, astringents herbs, bitters to restore digestion, and other herbs as needed, including nerve sedatives, anodynes, and enemas. Sixty-five different herbs were generally used by the Thomsonians (Berman 1954).

Disaffected with the elder Thomson's dictatorial and fanatical attitude, his movement split at its annual meeting in 1838. Coupled with the founder's death in 1843, this led to the decline and dissolution of the Thomsonian movement by the 1860s. Remnants of Thomsonian medicine survive in the pages of works like the ever-popular *Back to Eden* by Jethro Kloss, as well as the writings of the late Dr. John Christopher, whose popular herbal, *School of Natural Healing,* was in large measure responsible for the resurgence of interest in herbal self-medication in the United States during the 1970s.

Homeopathy, based on the medical theories developed by the German physician Samuel Hahnemann (1755–1843), in which infinitesimal or ultramolecular doses of a substance are administered to cure disease, emerged as a major medical modality in the United States during the 1840s. Homeopathy is based on the concept of "like cures like." That is, a substance that will produce a certain set of symptoms in a well person will also cure a matching symptom set in a diseased individual.

Botanic-medical groups, such as the Thomsonians, provided a clear economic threat to allopathic physicians. But the homeopaths, with rapidly growing numbers in the 1840s to 1860s and the strong support of the clergy, provided an even more formidable competition. Though homeopathy emerged in Europe in the late 1700s, it did not begin to become important in the United States until the 1840s. While Thomsonian physicians were largely self-taught, homeopathic physicians came largely from the ranks of orthodox medical practitioners.

A rallying cry emerged from the ranks of regular physicians in the 1830s calling for the "improvement of medical education." Various state and local allopathic medical societies called for the formation of a national association to address their collective needs and concerns. Many regional societies officially denounced the homeopaths as quacks. The perception of the introduction of "quackery" into their profession, as evidenced by declining medical education through conversion of physicians to homeopathy, led to the formation of the American Medical Association in 1846. Allopathic medicine was regarded with unprecedented contempt from the general population. Homeopathy was blamed for the decline in the physician's prestige (Coulter 1973).

Another group of medical practitioners flourished in the uncertain medical environment of nineteenth century America. They were known as the Eclectics. According to Harris Coulter, Wooster Beach (1794–1868), the acknowledged founder of Eclectic medicine, was driven by a Thomson-like hatred for allopathic physicians and an admiration for botanical remedies. Eclectic medicine began to evolve in the 1850s as Thomsonian medicine disappeared from the American medical scene. An Eclectic dispensatory was published in 1852, and passed through nineteen editions, the last published in 1909. By the 1880s, Eclectic medicine was as strong as homeopathy, with 10,000 practitioners nationwide. As many as eighteen Eclectic medical schools, many short-lived, had existed by the turn of the century. The major school, the Eclectic Medical Institute in Cincinnati, operated until 1939 (Coulter 1973, Berman 1954).

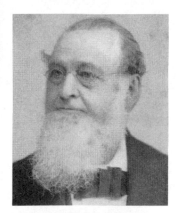

Professor John King, M.D.
at the age of 75

The major contribution of the Eclectics was the development of a pharmacy based on American medicinal plants. Two major personages emerge from the annals of Eclectic medicine. They are John King (1813–1893) and John Uri Lloyd (1849–1936).

John King, M.D., was a man of unusual abilities. By age nineteen King was proficient in five languages. He entered Wooster Beach's Reformed Medical College, graduating in 1838 when he was twenty-five years old. Dr. King began practicing medicine in New Bedford, Massachusetts, later moved to Kentucky, and finally settled in Cincinnati, Ohio, where he spent much of his professional career. He was coauthor (with R. S. Newton) of the *The Eclectic Dispensatory of the United States of America,* first published in 1852 (Felter 1902). Later editions became known as *King's American Dispensatory.* This work, still available as a reprint of the eighteenth edition (see Felter and Lloyd, 1898), remains one of the most useful reference works on American medicinal plants and clinical medical botany in general.

The gentle advice of Dr. King directed a young pharmacy apprentice, John Uri Lloyd, toward the development of pharmaceutical products derived from American medicinal plants for use by Eclectic physicians. Lloyd has been called "The Father of the American Materia Medica." As an individual, Lloyd represents the pinnacle of the accomplishments made by the Eclectic medical movement.

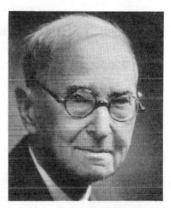

Lloyd became an apprentice in pharmacy at the age of fourteen. Eventually he went to work for H.M.

John Uri Lloyd at age 85

Merrell & Co., which manufactured medicines for use by Eclectic physicians. Lloyd and his two brothers, Curtis Gates Lloyd and Nelson Ashley Lloyd, later assumed ownership. The firm eventually became known as Lloyd Brothers Pharmacists, Inc. They manufactured 379 "specific medicines," primarily derived from American medicinal plants and made for the use of Eclectic practitioners. They were responsible for the first pharmaceutical preparations of Echinacea.

John Uri Lloyd was not just a manufacturing pharmacist. He

was a teacher, philanthropist, inventor, civic leader, and a prolific author. He authored more than 5000 periodical articles, six scientific treatises, eight scientific texts, sixty short stories, and eight novels. Perhaps best known is his novel *Etidorhpa* (1895), a metaphysical adventure which has been compared with the writings of Jules Verne, H. Rider Haggard, and Victor Hugo. He also won numerous professional awards and was perhaps one of the only medical personages of the nineteenth century to receive the respect of all factions of medical practitioners. J. U. Lloyd and his brothers also created the Lloyd Library and Museum in Cincinnati. Containing nearly a quarter million volumes, the Lloyd Library is to this day the world's most important medicinal plant library (Tyler and Tyler 1987).

John King and John Uri Lloyd are to be credited with the introduction of Echinacea to the medical profession. More on that subject will be presented in the chapter entitled "From Nostrum to Specific Medicine." For more information on the fascinating life of John Uri Lloyd see V.E. and V. M. Tyler (1987).

While the homeopaths and Eclectics flourished in the late nineteenth and early twentieth centuries, the allopathic physicians continued to strengthen their professional, legal, political, and economic gains. The AMA's Code of Ethics barred consultation with homeopaths and Eclectics. By the late nineteenth century an alliance was formed by the medical profession and the drug industry that influenced legislation to the exclusion of choices in medical care. In addition, the famous Flexner Report (A. Flexner 1910) produced by the Carnegie Endowment, in association with AMA's Council on Medical Education, represented the first national evaluation of medical schools. The findings, largely influenced by Nathan Colwell of the AMA, were adopted by many state examining boards. The net effect was that graduates of medical schools held in disfavor by the AMA, such as Eclectic and homeopathic medical schools, were not licensed to practice medicine. Eventually, the homeopathic and Eclectic medical schools met a forced demise (Coulter 1973).

The history of the past 150 years demonstrates that modern

medical practice in the United States, its drug laws, and its available pharmaceuticals are not necessarily, as might be assumed, products of a rational progression or the simple advancement of scientific achievement. Rather, they largely grow out of social, economic, and political factors that evolved out of the conflicts of the nineteenth century medical scene. This is not to debunk or discredit the contribution of modern medicine. Indeed, many major infectious diseases of the past have now been conquered. Emergency and surgical management of medical crises saves countless lives. Technology has provided diagnostic and treatment advances undreamed of just two decades ago. New and successful drugs have been developed to deal with many diseases. But, if the financial incentive for the development of new natural products were built into our drug laws, perhaps we could find safer natural compounds to replace the synthetic drugs now dominant. Evolution has better equipped the human race to deal with rational doses of preparations from natural sources than man-made chemicals, to which our genes have been exposed for only one generation (Foster and Duke 1990).

Along with the dramatic improvements in medical care have come dramatic and rapidly spiraling cost increases. The public is looking for alternatives. Osteopathy and chiropractic care are widely available. Still, naturopathy (which borrows some elements from the Eclectic tradition), acupuncture, and homeopathy are available only in isolated enclaves. The public is becoming increasingly dissatisfied with allopathic medical care and its costs. Despite advances in modern medicine, AIDS, the 200 or more diseases lumped into the category of cancer, and even the common cold are still a challenge to modern medicine.

The answers, in part, lie in a social, economic, and legal restructuring of the health care system which would stimulate competition even among small manufacturers. I believe we need a system that stimulates basic research, rewarded by scientific advancement rather than by patents. A system that allows freedom of choice for the patient. A system that stimulates broad interaction and referral among appropriate medical modalities rather than exclusion and monopoly. Are such ideas pipe dreams, or will they be realized as the inevitable outcome of the cyclic, rational evolution of medicine? Time will tell.

The time has come for a melding of technological Western medicine and the use of herbs in health care. One major factor that has prevented herbalism and modern Western medicine from moving forward in the United States is the historical medical antagonism and schism that has here existed for a full two centuries. Perceived nonscientific or nonaccepted aspects of herbalism and the use of plant-derived drugs in conventional therapy must find a happy medium where progress can move forward for the benefit of all.

Plant drugs have been emerging as an important element of health care worldwide. This is particularly true in China, where over the past forty years considerable resources have been devoted to understanding the efficacy of herb use in traditional Chinese medicine through extensive chemical, pharmacological, and clinical studies. In the case of many herbal remedies, this research has established a scientific basis for the traditional applications of herbs.

In Germany, the use of preparations of whole plants or plant principles is called phytotherapy. Herb products, standardized to predictable amounts of the crude herb or isolated plant principles, are called phytopharmaceuticals. In Europe, phytotherapy has emerged as a distinct, accepted scientific discipline (Weiss 1985). To be accepted in modern health care, herbs must be subjected to scientific scrutiny. I believe a major starting point for scientific investigation is studying the use of herbs for the treatment of disease in a historical or traditional context. Science is necessary for the the progress and future development of herbal medicine. The melding of the valuable aspects of traditional herbal wisdom and their application to modern health care are mutually inclusive, not mutually exclusive.

We are at the threshold of a new era of natural products research. The negative vestiges of bygone antagonisms should give rise to new applications of herbal medicine to public health care. A rational change in our drug laws as they relate to the development and labeling of natural products is essential. So, too, is a shift in the attitude of those who perceive themselves as sitting on opposite sides of an invisible fence. When viewed with objectivity and an open, inquiring mind, Echinacea symbolizes the potential of the new herbalism, where science and tradition can be blended to produce positive results.

Understanding How Echinacea is Used

Since the 1970s there has been a growing trend toward people taking more responsibility for their own health. Interest in diet, exercise, and relaxation has become an integral part of daily existence. We live in times of increased stress, both physically and psychically. That stress, be it from environmental pollutants, overwork, or a myriad of other factors induced by modern living, may result in becoming more susceptible to catching a cold or flu. It could adversely affect the immune system, causing more serious chronic diseases. The AIDS crisis has heightened our awareness of our immune systems. If our immune system fails, as it does in full-blown development of the HIV infection, the end result is tragically fatal.

Immunology is such a rapidly growing field that even specialists in immune system research have a difficult time keeping up with the field's advances. We are only beginning to understand the broad functions of the immune system in maintaining health, dealing with minor and common ailments, or in combating chronic disease. The immune system basically helps to balance the internal functions of the body with the external environment. It does so by a number of mechanisms. Immune system responses include the highly selective response of specific resistance against specific microorganisms by antibodies and other mechanisms. Nonspecific immune resistance, however, helps the body deal with any foreign substance. This resistance may include responses of the mucous membranes and skin, inflammation, fever, and other factors such as phagocytosis by cells such as the white blood cells, which devour foreign invaders. Specific immune resistance includes cell-mediated immune response, in which specialized cells, such as T-cells, that are specific to a recognized antigen, migrate to the site of a foreign invader and destroy it or cause other cells to destroy it (Halstead and Hood 1984).

The immune system stimulating activity of Echinacea involves mechanisms of both specific and nonspecific immune responses. The details on its action are found in chapter 4, "Modern Research and Future Potential." Echinacea works with the immune system to help prevent minor ailments such as colds and flu. Future research may provide new applications. At this point, it should be made clear that the term "immunostimulant," as applied to Echinacea, does not imply that it is in any way useful for chronic disease such as cancer or AIDS. It is important that the use of Echinacea be understood in proper context.

There is a long tradition of thought regarding the stimulation of nonspecific defense mechanisms in the human body in traditional medicine, though not in those terms. Examples are the superior tonics of traditional Chinese medicine, such as Astragalus *(Huang-qi)* and Ginseng *(Panax* spp.). Recent research has confirmed a rational scientific basis for the use of these and other Chinese herbs in helping to balance the immune system. In Germany, the concept of "general reorientation or returning to health of the organism as a whole" is known as *Umstimmungstherapie.* This concept is employed as an alternative to conventional therapies, as well as a prophylaxis or preventive against infections, especially when the immune system must be activated under situations involving impaired immune response. Such situations may include infectious disease, multiple infections, persistent infections, or chronic infections. Another application is the prevention of opportunistic infections of patients at risk, especially viral infections (Wagner and Proksch 1985).

In West Germany, Echinacea products are used as a general nonspecific stimulant to the immune system, helping to support and stabilize cellular immunity for the prevention and treatment of infections. Echinacea salves are used for hard to heal wounds and sores, inflammatory skin diseases such as eczema, minor burns, sunburn, and as a topical application to herpes sores (Herpes simplex). Liquid extracts and tinctures are used as a preventive for colds, flu, infections, psoriasis, to treat viral-induced canker sores, and to support long-term treatments with antibiotics.

Injectable forms of the drug, administered by physicians, have been used in a wide range of clinical applications, including polyarthritis, tonsillitis, infections of the urogenital tract, allergies, and gynecological infections. Injectable forms are considered fast acting and are used by European physicians primarily for severe conditions.

The oral dosage forms, such as extracts and tinctures, are documented as safe when used in normal dosage and act more slowly. They are sold in health and natural food outlets in the United States and a variety of retail outlets in Europe. They help to enhance resistance to infection, stimulate the lymphatic vascular system, and stimulate fibroblasts (cells involved in the development of connective tissue). Used primarily to enhance or "stimulate" the body's own resistance against infections, oral dosages are most widely used to prevent colds and flu. If taken at the onset of symptoms in small frequent doses, every two to three hours for the first two or three days, the herb often helps to mobilize the body's own resistance to the condition (Weiss 1985).

Many herbs that were once referred to as blood purifiers or "alteratives" are sometimes termed "immunostimulants." Echinacea is probably the most widely used immune system-stimulating herb product in West Germany.

Since 1950, over 200 papers have been published on the chemistry, pharmacology, and clinical applications of Echinacea. Most of them are published in German scientific journals.

How to Use this Book

Echinacea: Nature's Immune Enhancer provides a comprehensive look at this important plant group. The chapters are arranged so that you may read sections that interest you, or refer to them as needed. Sources of information are referenced throughout, allowing the reader to seek the original reference, if desired. Remember, most libraries are linked by computer. The interlibrary loan system in essence makes all libraries one library. While many of the references are obscure, if you wish to find original source materials they can usually be obtained within a few weeks. The titles of foreign-language scientific periodical articles have generally been excluded from the bibliography. English-language article citations include the article name.

Native groups of the Great Plains used Echinacea for more purposes than any other medicinal plant. You will find details on American Indian usage in the first chapter. Current use and interest in Echinacea is a direct result of native American wisdom.

The second and third chapters explore the controversial medical history of Echinacea use among Europeans and European settlers. The story begins in the 1760s and culminates in the 1930s with the widespread use of the plant among Eclectic medical practitioners. Chapter 4, "Modern Research and Future Potential," reviews the scientific literature since 1939, explaining how Echinacea is used. Chapters 5 and 6 discuss ways Echinacea is prepared and safety issues.

Like many medicinal plants, several Echinacea species are extractively harvested from wild habitats without regard for their sustainability. If Echinacea is to be widely used, it must be grown commercially. Chapter 7 gives propagation and cultivation information for the farm and garden.

The importance of proper identity, correct use of names, and accurate labeling is disclosed in chapter 8, on substitution and adulteration—a surprising story of mistaken identity. Research on Echinacea's potential as an insecticide is discussed in chapter 9.

Chapters 10 through 13 present information on Echinacea's chemical components, the taxonomic evolution of its botanical names, its botanical characteristics, and identification and distribution. With chapter 14, the most important message is saved for last—the need for conservation of wild Echinacea populations.

The appendix is a resource section of where you may purchase

Echinacea seeds and plants. Finally, we provide an extensive bibliography of references from both past and present.

Echinacea: Nature's Immune Enhancer is aimed at all persons, lay or scientist, with an interest in the genus in hopes that it will contribute to our understanding of this fascinating plant group, its history, and uses. We also hope it sparks serious interest in commercial cultivation of Echinacea, as well as interest among home gardeners, so as to encourage preservation of wild populations. Overharvesting poses a serious threat to the genetic diversity of Echinacea, as the genus becomes, as John Uri Lloyd predicted, "ardently sought and widely used."

1

The Universal Remedy of the Plains Indians

Ethnobotanical Aspects

American Indian groups of the Great Plains and adjacent regions used Echinacea for many purposes. The study of the use of plants among indigenous peoples is known as ethnobotany. Ethnobotanical data on Echinacea was collected only after the native groups that used it were driven onto reservations. Therefore, the ethnobotany of Echinacea is fragmentary at best. However, from what is known about native American uses of Echinacea, it was obviously one of the most important native medicinal plants—used for everything from colds to cancers.

The founder of the world's first ethnobotanical laboratory, Melvin R. Gilmore, noted the importance of Echinacea to native groups of the Missouri River Region. "This plant was universally used as an antidote for snake bite and other venomous bites and stings and poisonous conditions. Echinacea seems to have been used as a remedy for more ailments than any other plant" (Gilmore 1919, p. 131).

Medicinal uses for *E. angustifolia* were many and varied. The Omaha-Ponca used *E. angustifolia* for a wide range of purposes. The whole root was placed on toothaches until the pain subsided and was used on enlarged glands (like mumps). A smoke fumigant of Echinacea was used to treat headaches in people and distemper in horses. It was also used for snakebites, stings, and other poisonous conditions. Externally, the juice of the root was used to bathe burns

20

and make the intense heat of a sweat lodge more bearable. Jugglers were said to have bathed their arms and hands in the juice of the plant so that they could take a piece of meat from a boiling pot with their bare hands without experiencing pain. A Winnebago Indian told Melvin Gilmore that he used the plant to make his mouth insensible to heat so he could put a live coal in his mouth for show. The Oglala Dakota used the root of *E. pallida* internally for toothache and bad colds (Gilmore 1913a, 1913b, 1919). Wolf Chief, a Hidatsu, reported a warrior would chew a small piece of *E. pallida* root as a stimulant when traveling at night (Nickel 1974).

The Cheyenne employed an infusion of the powdered leaves and roots for sore throat, gums, and mouth. They also chewed the roots for the same ailments. For sore throat, the whole root was chewed, letting the saliva run down the throat to sooth the irritation. The juice of the root was placed in the mouth to relieve the ache of a hollow tooth. An infusion of the root and leaves was rubbed on a sore neck to relieve pain (Grinnell 1923). The root has been chewed to stimulate saliva and assuage thirst, especially for participants of the sun dance (Hart 1981). The root tea is drunk as a treatment for arthritis, measles, mumps, rheumatism, and smallpox. Mixed with *Lycopodium* spores and skunk oil, the mashed root was applied to boils after lancing (Kindscher 1989).

Like the Cheyenne and many other native groups, the Crow chewed the fresh root to allay the pain of toothaches. A juice from the roots was used for colds and the treatment of colic (Toineeta 1970). The Comanche used the root of Echinacea species for toothache and sore throat. For sore throat, the root was decocted. The root itself was held against an aching tooth (Carlson and Jones 1939).

The Meskwaki used the root in medicines for relieving stomach cramps, eczema, and fits. H. H. Smith (1928) notes that one polyherbal combination in the Volney Jones collection, termed "potatcigan," included *E. angustifolia* (or *E. pallida*) in combination with *Asarum canadense*, *Euphorbia collata*, and *Monarda punctata*. The mixture was used to treat stomach cramps. Smith's informant, John McIntosh (Kepeosatok), actually a Prairie

Potawatomi married to a Meskwaki who spent most of his time on the Meskwaki Reservation in Tama, Iowa, included the root of *E. angustifolia,* the root *Verbena hastata,* and a yellow root from Cedar Falls, Iowa, (described by Smith as "probably" *Jeffersonia diphylla*) in a prescription for eczema.

In addition to using the root for snakebites, the Sioux used the fresh root of *E. angustifolia* to treat hydrophobia (rabies) and septic conditions (Smith 1928). The Pawnee utilized the root for rattle-snake bite (Wedel 1936). In Montana, at the western edge of its range, it was also used as an antidote to rattlesnake bite (Blankenship 1905). *Echinacea angustifolia* root was used by the Lakota to treat toothache, tonsillitis, and pain in the bowels (Munson 1981). Kindscher (1989), in traveling to the Rosebud Reservation in 1987, observed that the Purple Coneflower is still widely harvested and used for a variety of medicinal purposes.

The Kiowa chewed the ground root and slowly swallowed the juice for the treatment of coughs and sore throat. Vestal and Schultes (1939) note that the Kiowa use of the root as a cough medicine dates from early times and is not reported for other tribes. T. N. Campbell (1951) quotes notations from the herbarium specimens of Gideon Lincecum, a self-taught physician who lived in eastern Mississippi near Choctaw territory from 1818–1848. Lincecum's herbarium of 305 pressed-plant specimens is housed in the library of the University of Texas at Austin. Lincecum recorded the use of *E. purpurea* for coughs. "The tincture of the roots of this plant has been used with success in bad cough, and dyspepsis attended with a bad cough. . . . The Choctaws use it for the above purposes, by chewing and swallowing the saliva. They keep a small piece of the root in the mouth nearly all the time, continuing its use for a long time" (Campbell 1951, p. 288).

Hartwell (1969, p. 139), citing the central files of the National Cancer Institute, notes Indian use of *E. angustifolia* and *E. pallida* in breast cancer, with "over 100 cases 'cured.' "

It is possible that some of the uses reported above for *E. angustifolia* were in fact for *E. pallida,* since several of the native peoples who utilized the plant group lived in the range of *E. pallida*. It is also probable that the two species were used interchangeably.

The Omaha distinguished Echinacea as *nu* (male), and *wa-u* (female), the apparent difference being between root size, the *nu* being larger, and the *wa-u* smaller. The *wa-u* was considered the more effective medicine (Gilmore 1909, p. 21). (In Gilmore 1913a, the male is listed as *nuga* and the female as *miga*.) It could be conjectured that these distinctions were made between *E. pallida* and *E. angustifolia*. The principal historical home of the Omaha is along the Missouri River in northeastern Nebraska. In eastern Nebraska, *E. angustifolia* var. *angustifolia* takes on an intermediate form, with characteristics similar to *E. pallida* (McGregor 1968a). Perhaps this intermediate series accounts for the Omaha's *nu (nuga)*, with the more western *E. angustifolia* var. *angustifolia* populations of smaller plants accounting for the higher quality *wa-u (miga)*.

E. purpurea was used by the Delaware for advanced venereal disease (Tantaquidgeon 1942).

Dr. F. V. Hayden noted the use of *E. purpurea*, though the species was probably misrepresented. The reference more likely refers to *E. angustifolia* or *E. pallida:* "Purple cone flower: called Rattlesnake weed in the west . . . is found abundantly throughout the country. Root very pungent. Used very effectively by the traders and Indians for the cure of the bite of the rattlesnake" (1859, p. 738).

In addition to a multitude of medicinal uses for fresh and dried roots and leaves of several Echinacea species, the dried flower heads were used by tribes of the Missouri River region, the Meskwaki, and the Kiowa as hair combs. Children of the Pawnee used the dried flower stalks for a game in which two stalks were whirled around one another. One Pawnee name for the plant, *ksapitahako*, (*iksa*, a hand, and *pitahako*, to whirl) refers to this child's play. *Saparidukahts*, another Pawnee name for the plant, meaning mushroom medicine, apparently refers to the similarity of the shape of the Echinacea flower head compared to a mushroom. The Omaha-Ponca called the plant *mika-hi*, meaning comb plant, or *ikigahai*, meaning to comb. Another Omaha name refers to the use of the plant to treat sore eyes. The Dakota called it *ichalipe-hu* — "whip plant" (Gilmore 1919). *Wetop,* a Meskwaki name, translates to "widow's comb." Another Meskwaki name, *ashosikwimia'kuk,* means "smells like a muskrat scent" (Smith 1928). The Kiowa called the plant *dain-pai-a* and *awdl-son-a* (Vestal and Schultes 1939).

Obviously, Echinacea was an important medicinal plant among native peoples of North America, but that fact was lost upon European settlers until well into the nineteenth century. The traditional native wisdom of Echinacea's medicinal use sets the stage for the development of the plant's use in a historical Western herbal context, as well as its development as a modern phytopharmaceutical. The story of its introduction into Western medical practice follows.

2
From Nostrum to Specific Medicine

Echinacea was not introduced under authoritative auspices, such as might establish it in the practice of physicians generally. On the contrary, its origin as a constituent of a "home cure" remedy made by an illiterate, unknown physician, was used as an argument to authoritatively condemn it.

J. U. Lloyd (1924, p. 15)

Medical History of Echinacea: the American Experience

As was the case with most American medicinal plants, the early European settlers learned of the uses of Echinacea from the Indians. Echinacea species were popularly known as Indian Head, Scurvy Root, Black Sampson, Niggerhead, Comb Flower, Hedgehog, Red Sunflower, Purple Coneflower, Missouri Snake-root, Kansas Snakeroot, Rattlesnake Weed and, in the Ozarks, as Droops, referring to the reflexed ray flowers of *E. pallida*. References to the use of Echinacea were sparse until the late nineteenth century.

Johann David Schöpf, in *Materia Medica Americana* (1787), widely regarded as the earliest scholarly work on American medicinal plants, citing Clayton, mentions the use of *Echinacea purpurea* for treating ulcers caused by saddles on a horse's back.

The younger John Clayton (1693–1773) was one of the earliest explorers of Virginia's native plants. He should not to be confused with his father, the senior John Clayton, an early Crown-appointed attorney general of Virginia, or his older distant cousin, John Clayton, an English clergyman who spent several years in Virginia in the late 1600s. Our John Clayton had sent plant specimens, seeds, and a catalog of plants he found in Virginia to Johann Frederick Gronovius (1690–1762), a physician and naturalist in Leiden. To Clayton's dismay, in 1739 Gronovius published Clayton's "catalog" as *Flora Virginica,* but without Clayton's permission. One of the plants included was *E. purpurea.*

Christopher Hobbs (1989) cites Gronovius's *Flora Virginica* as the earliest reference to medicinal uses of Echinacea. However, the comment on medicinal uses, extracted by Hobbs from Berkeley and Berkeley (1963), does not appear in the 1739 edition of *Flora Virginicus.* Rather, it appears in the expanded 1762 second edition, published by Gronovius's son, Laurens Theodoor Gronovius (1730–1773). This work was published in the same year that the elder Gronovius died. It is the second edition of *Flora Virginicus* that is quoted by Schöpf. The earliest known reference to medicinal use of an Echinacea species would therefore seem to have been made in 1762. The notes of Clayton are cited by the younger Gronovius as the source of the information.

Until the 1880s, additional mention of medicinal use of Echinacea in the literature is rare. The controversial nineteenth-century naturalist C. S. Rafinesque (1783–1840) who was often described as "gifted and erratic," lists *E. purpurea* under a generic name of his own creation: *Helichroa.* The root is "acrid and burning, used in syphilis by the Mandan; Schoepf says to cure the ulcers on the back of horses" (Rafinesque 1830, vol. II, p. 227).

John L. Riddle, a Louisiana physician best known as the inventor of the binocular microscope, notes that the root of *E. purpurea* is aromatic and carminative (1835, p. 500).

The eminent American botanist Asa Gray, who trained as a medical doctor and later became known as "the father of American botany," occasionally noted medicinal plant usage in early editions of his *Manual of Botany.* The first edition notes that *Echinaea purpurea* (as *Rudbeckia purpurea*) has a "thick [root], black, very pungent to the taste, used in popular medicine under the name of Black Sampson" (Gray 1848, p. 223). Despite his medical training, Gray's interest in medicinal usage of the plant seems to go little beyond recording the colloquial name. It was called "Black Sampson by the quack doctors," he wrote in a later work (Gray 1870, p. 205).

In 1852 *E. purpurea* was mentioned in the literature by both Eclectic physicians and allopathic physicians ("regular" doctors). A note on the medicinal uses of *E. purpurea* appears in the first edition of John King's *Eclectic Dispensatory* under an article on thimbleweed *(Rudbeckia lacinata)*. "The *Rudbeckia Purpurea,* or red sunflower, is said to be used with benefit in syphilis; the root is the part employed, and which, when fresh, is acrid and burning" (King and Newton 1852, p. 351).

In the same year, Dr. A. Clapp also mentioned the medicinal uses of *E. purpurea* in his "Report on Medical Botany" in the *Transactions of the American Medical Association.* Clapp described the root as aromatic and carminative, and noted that it was used in popular medicine.

The first use mentioned in the literature is for the treatment of sores on horses (Gronovius 1762). Other veterinary uses were also recorded. Dr. J. S. Leachman of Sharon, Oklahoma, writing in the October 1914 issue of the *The Gleaner,* states, "Old settlers all believe firmly in the virtues of Echinacea root, and use it as an aid in nearly every sickness. If a cow or horse does not eat well, the people administer Echinacea, cut up and put in feed. I have noticed that puny stock treated in this manner soon begin to thrive" (Lloyd 1924, p. 18).

These are relatively obscure, mostly passing references to Echinacea. When it comes to the medical history of Echinacea and its introduction into widespread use, two names stand prominently— John Uri Lloyd and John King, both of Cincinnati, as mentioned in the introduction. To reiterate, John Uri Lloyd, a pharmacist, was one of the leading proponents of the use and development of American medicinal plants. He served as president of the American Pharmaceutical Association (1887–88), and founded Lloyd Brothers Pharmacists, Inc., a manufacturing firm specializing in preparations made from American medicinal plants. In addition to authoring over 5,000 scientific papers, Lloyd wrote eight novels and several books on American medicinal plants, including his monumental *Drugs & Medicine of North America* (2 vols.), coauthored by his younger brother and partner, Curtis Gates Lloyd, a botanist and renowned mycologist. One of the Lloyd Brothers' greatest lasting achievements was the establishment of the Lloyd Library and Museum in Cincinnati, the world's most important pharmacognosy library. *Lloydia* (now the *Journal of Natural Products)* was named in honor of the Lloyds (Simons 1972).

John King was one of the most prominent Eclectic medical practitioners of the last century. In addition to authoring the *Eclectic Dispensatory,* in print for over sixty years and recently reprinted, King is credited with bringing the medicinal uses of Echinacea to light and discovering podophyllin from the Mayapple *(Podophyllum peltatum.)*

According to J. U. Lloyd in his *Treatise on Echinacea* (1924), *E. angustifolia* was not introduced to the medical profession until 1887. It was a "quack" doctor, a purveyor of nostrums, Dr. H. C. F. Meyer of Pawnee City, Nebraska, who first brought Echinacea to

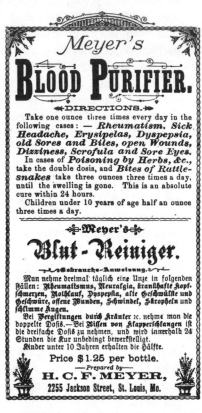

Meyer's Blood Purifier, the first Echinacea product

the attention of John King and J. U. Lloyd. For sixteen years, Meyer had been marketing his secret proprietary formula, "Meyer's Blood Purifier," which contained, among other ingredients, hops, wormwood, and Echinacea. Although Meyer had used Echinacea root in his medicine for years, he did not know of the identity of the plant, having supposedly learned of its uses from the Indians.

In 1885, Meyer sent root samples of *E. angustifolia* to John Uri Lloyd and samples of his blood purifier to Dr. King, in hopes that they would endorse his product and offer it for sale to the medical community. King, of course, was unwilling to endorse a secret formula that didn't even list the ingredients on the label. That was the mark of so-called patent medicines, which in fact were not patented. To patent them, their maker had to disclose the ingredients.

Lloyd replied that he would be unable to identify the plant from the root alone, and that his company Lloyd Brothers, Pharmacists, Inc., could only introduce a new drug under its proper botanical name. On June 7, 1886, Meyer sent the dried whole plant to Lloyd. Curtis Gates Lloyd identified the plant as *E. angustifolia*.

Meyer made extravagant claims for his product. The back label of Meyer's Blood Purifier read:

Take one ounce three times everyday in the following cases: Rheumatism, Sick Headache, Erysipelas, Dyspepsia, Old Sores, and Biles, Open Wounds, Dizziness, Scrofula, and Sore Eyes. In case of Poisoning by Herbs & C., take the double dosis, and Bites of Rattlesnakes take three ounces three times a day until the swelling is gone. This is an absolute cure within 24 hours (Lloyd 1924).

After the identification of the plant by C.G. Lloyd, Meyer's new label read:

This is a powerful drug as an Alterative and Antiseptic in all tumorous and Syphilitic indications; old chronic sores, such as fever sores, old ulcers, Carbuncles, Piles, eczema, wet or dry, can be cured quick and active; also Erysipelas. It will not fail in gangrene. In fever it is a specific; typhoid can be adverted in two to three days; also in Malaria, Malignant Remittent and Mountain fever it is a specific. It relieves pain, swelling, inflammation, by local use, internal and external. It has not and will not fail to cure Diphtheria quick. It cures bites from the bee to the rattlesnake, it is a specific. Has been tested in more than fifty cases of mad dog bites in humans and in every case it prevented hydrophobia. It has cured hydrophobia. It is perfectly harmless, internal and external. Dose—One half to one fluid-drachm 3 or 4 times a day" (Lloyd 1924, p. 16).

Meyer was so confident in his claims that he offered to come to Cincinnati, and—before Dr. King and J. U. Lloyd—allow himself to be bitten by several rattlesnakes, to prove the truth of his claims. Lloyd and King naturally declined the offer. Meyer claimed to know of over 600 cases in which his remedy had not failed to cure rattlesnake bites.

Yet such a broad number of extravagant claims, "strongly prejudiced me against it," wrote J. U. Lloyd (1924, p. 3). "However Dr. King, with his usual thoughtfulness, consideration, and care proposed to investigate the matter, and from the drug forwarded by Dr. Meyer I at once made for Dr. King several specimens of liquid preparations and then I passed the subject from my mind as one among a multitude of such before me, destined to remain in obscurity" (1904a, p. 11).

Several months passed before Lloyd heard from King regarding his experiments with Echinacea. Finally, King instructed Lloyd to send Echinacea preparations to a number of leading Eclectic physicians for further trials, including Dr. I. J. M. Goss of Atlanta, Dr. H.T. Webster of Oakland, California, and others. King had become convinced of the remedy's value.

Two years after beginning to investigate *E. angustifolia* King introduced the plant to Eclectic practitioners. ". . . It will be observed from what follows that he [Dr. Meyer] entertains a very exalted idea of his discovery, which certainly merits a careful investigation by our practitioners; and should it be found to contain only one-half the virtues he attributes to it, it will form an important addition to our materia medica — one for which the profession, as well as the afflicted, will ever be under indebtedness to him . . ." (King 1887, p. 79).

Lloyd's skepticism persisted. "All of this time, I was rather resisting the claims made by the enthusiastic friends of *E. angustifolia,* believing that conservatism is to be preferred to over-enthusiasm" (1904a, p. 12).

However, soon after the appearance of King's 1887 article, Lloyd Brothers Pharmacists, Inc. made Echinacea preparations available to the medical profession. Lloyd conceded:

> Owing to what this writer now views as inexcusable conservatism, he persistently refused to introduce and distribute any Echinacea preparation until some time after Dr. King had reported favorably concerning the action of the drug, both in his home in the treatment of Mrs. King, and in general practice. . . .
>
> My own delay in its general introduction is to me now a subject of self-criticism. I am now more pronouncedly of the opinion, as experiences multiply, that a person who is restricted to laboratory experiments, especially if he be more or less adversely prejudiced (as I was against Echinacea), is not in a position to judge with discretion. Nor is a laboratory man to be considered as "authority" in clinical directions which applies no less forcibly to inadequate drugs *introduced* under laboratory propaganda than to those *worthy* decried thereby (1924, p. 11–12).

Lloyd wholly credits Dr. King's confidence in Echinacea as responsible for its introduction to the medical community. Perhaps the most convincing test for Echinacea came in King's own home. His wife had suffered from a "virulent cancer" for many years. King had tried a large number of remedies to relieve her symptoms, with little success. Finally he resorted to Echinacea, which both he and Mrs. King claimed produced her only relief. Mrs. King told J. U. Lloyd that whenever she stopped using Echinacea her symptoms intensified. Until the day she died, she could not be without Echinacea.

Following King's original endorsement of *E. angustifolia,* its popularity grew rapidly among Eclectic practitioners. Dr. H. T. Webster wrote an extensive account of the therapeutic uses of the plant in his *Dynamical Therapeutics,* a standard text of Eclectic physicians. In 1888, a Dr. Goss of Chicago praised the remedy in mad dog bites, chronic catarrh, chronic ulcers, gonorrhea, and syphilis. Dr. A. Parker of Wilbur, Nebraska, reported success in using Echinacea to treat a case of "hopeless" blood poisoning.

Harvey Wickes Felter, another prominent Eclectic physician and a collaborator with J. U. Lloyd in the later editions of *King's Eclectic Dispensatory,* included it among the most important Eclectic contributions.

> Conspicuous among the remedies introduced within recent years, Echinacea undoubtedly takes the first rank. . . . As with all new remedies, it has suffered the usual over-estimating, in that it has been endorsed for almost the whole range of human ailments. . . . Many over-sanguine statements concerning its wonderful—yes, practically impossible—virtues have, however, been judiciously withheld from publication, lest a remedy of great value should be placed in bad repute through exaggerated reports, a condition that has not been altogether avoided (1898, p. 79).

It was not only the various and extravagant claims that prejudiced some physicians against Echinacea, but the person who discovered its properties as well. Dr. H. C. F. Meyer was an unschooled, self-made physician. His remedy was immediately dismissed in some circles as a quack remedy. Dr. King, though a medical doctor highly respected for his skills, was an "irregular" doctor, a follower of the Eclectic school.

In large part the Eclectics were considered quacks (as well as competitors) by the "regular"or allopathic physicians. The Eclectics were constantly attacking the regular medical doctors for their use of dangerous mineral remedies such as mercury preparations, while the the regular physicians where constantly attacking the Eclectics for using drugs they deemed worthless. If a new drug was introduced by one group, inevitably the other attacked it. Despite the quarrels, both groups heavily relied upon American medicinal plants.

In response to a letter requesting, "Kindly inform me as the the real properties of Echinacea," the editor of the *Journal of the American Medical Association (JAMA)* discredited Echinacea in the February 27, 1909, issue. "Echinacea has been claimed to have anesthetic, sialagogue, antiseptic, diaphoretic, alterative, and several other properties. Like many other discarded drugs, it has failed to sustain the reputation give by its enthusiasts years ago; it is now seldom prescribed under its own name. In common with numerous other little-used drugs, it is finding a place in proprietary mixtures, whose manufacturers make use of the early enthusiastic and unverified reports to endow their nostrums with remarkable therapeutic properties" (pp. 720–721).

The AMA's Council on Pharmacy and Chemistry published a report, "Echinacea Considered Valueless," in the November 27, 1909, *JAMA*. "It is worth noticing—although it is not surprising—that these far-reaching claims have been made on no better basis than that of clinical trials by unknown men who have not otherwise achieved any general reputation as acute, discriminating, and reliable observers. . . . In lack of any scientific scrutiny of claims made for it, Echinacea is deemed unworthy of further consideration until more evidence is presented in its favor" (p. 1836).

A study conducted by James F. Couch and Leigh T. Giltner, USDA Pathological Division, Bureau of Animal Industry (1920) drew similar conclusions. The report, "An Experimental Study of Echinacea Therapy," investigated the effects of several preparations including Lloyd Brother's Specific Medicine Echinacea, a fluid extract of Echinacea, Echinacea tincture, and Subculoyd Inula (Elecampane) and Echinacea on guinea pigs infected with tetanus, septicemia, anthrax, dried powdered rattlesnake venin, tuberculosis, and trypanosomiasis. The report concluded that, "in none of the diseases treated with Echinacea, was any evidence obtained to show that the plant exerts any influence upon the course of infectious process under laboratory conditions. . . . It does not appear, therefore, that Echinacea or the preparations of Inula and Echinacea are of value in the treatment of diseases produced by microorganisms and their toxic products" (Couch and Giltner 1920, p. 67).

However, James H. Beal's comments (1921) on Couch and Giltner's paper suggests that completely different conclusions can be drawn from the results. Beal takes each experiment on a case by case basis, and in each instance but one points out that while Couch and Giltner found Echinacea and its preparations of no value, if the same experimental results were viewed from a clinician's eyes (rather than those of a laboratory researcher), it would be fair to conclude that the Echinacea preparations were in fact valuable.

"While these experiments of Couch and Giltner are perhaps too few in number to be regarded as conclusive, they are of very great value as illustrating the difference in the viewpoints and methods of deduction of the laboratory worker and of the clinician, a difference that may lead to diametrically opposed conclusions from the same observed facts" (Beal 1921, p. 232).

Despite the AMA and USDA denunciations of Echinacea and those who used it, its use grew. Case reports and verbal commendation of clinical success with the plant made it one of the most widely used American medicinal plants of the late nineteenth and early twentieth centuries. By 1921, Echinacea and its preparations became the most widely sold medicines from an American medicinal plant. Out of 239 Specific Medicines made from the indigenous materia medica by the Lloyd Brothers, Echinacea outsold the second most popular remedy, *Chionanthus,* by more than two to one. It should be noted that Lloyd Brother's Specific Medicines were sold only to medical practitioners and not to the general public.

3

Medicinal Uses of Echinacea by Eclectic Physicians

Diseases and conditions for which Echinacea was employed by Eclectics were many and varied. The label of Lloyd Brothers' "Specific Medicine Echinacea" stated that it was "an alterative of great value in strumous diathesis, syphilis, old sores, and wounds. A powerful antiseptic, locally and internally, in diphtheria, typhoid conditions, cholera infantum, and blood poisoning."

J. U. Lloyd (1924, p. 13)

H.W. Felter felt that qualifying terms such as antiseptic and alterative did little to convey with accuracy the virtues of Echinacea. "The day is rapidly approaching when these qualifying terms will have no place in medicine," he predicted, "especially so with regard to such terms as alterative, stimulant, tonic, etc. . . . If any single statement could be made concerning the virtues of Echinacea it would read something like this, 'A corrector of the depravation of the body's fluids;' and even this does not sufficiently cover the ground" (Felter 1898, p. 84).

Felter contended that the main action of Echinacea was in balancing changes in body fluids produced by either internal or external causes. Boils, carbuncles, abscesses, and inflammation of glands caused by venom, diphtheria, cerebrospinal meningitis, "bad blood," and attendant weakness or loss of strength could effectively be dealt with using Echinacea preparations. Many reports of Echinacea's efficacy are found in cases of blood poisoning. A hand crushed and thought in need of amputation was saved by Echinacea, despite the hand's striking gangrenous condition.

Some nineteenth-century physicians reported that Echinacea was useful against cancerous growths, particularly of the mucous membranes. Echafolta, a concentrated preparation of the root excluding most sugar compounds, chlorophyll, and coloring matter (manufactured by Lloyd Brothers), was reported to overcome the odors of some carcinomas. It was used in cancerous cachexia. One physician reported that a case of breast cancer was long held in check with Echinacea.

Echinacea was reportedly used to mitigate the pain and inflammation of gonorrhea and syphilis. Dr. Snyder extolled Echinacea as an effective remedy for impotence. Skin disorders such as eczema, psoriasis, acne, and poison ivy responded favorably to treatment with Echinacea. It was used to lessen pain and inflammation of tonsillitis. Echinacea has been recommended as an appetizer to improve digestion, quiet dyspepsia, and calm intestinal indigestion. It has been called very effective in ulcerative stomatitis, as well.

Finley Ellingwood, M. D., (1914), an important Eclectic physician, professor, and author, recommended Echinacea tincture as a local anesthetic, producing a burning sensation at first (because of the alcohol in tinctures) followed by "entire relief of pain in many cases."

Ellingwood counts among Echinacea's effects a stimulation of the lymphatic system as well as improved digestion in the stomach and the bowels. He suggested it also stimulates circulation, liver function, and nerve tone. He recommended its use in nettle stings, scorpion stings, and suggested that it may be useful in strychnine poisoning, in addition to the usual complement of diseases for which Eclectics employed Echinacea.

Another New York Eclectic physician, Dr. A. M. Liebstein, called *E. angustifolia* "The king of plant remedies influencing the character of the blood, and the leading alterative in the entire materia medica." Liebstein claimed that Echinacea greatly improved endocrine function, stimulated capillary circulation and respiration, and had a beneficial effect on the sympathetic nervous system (Liebstein 1927, p. 316).

From the earliest ethnobotanical references, the use of Echinacea in treatment of snakebites was listed among its qualities. In his first article on *E. angustifolia,* King quotes H. C. F. Meyer on the effect of Echinacea on snake bites. "I injected some of the (rattlesnake) poison into my system, on the first finger of the left hand; the swelling was rapid, and in six hours was up to my elbow. At this time I took a dose of the medicine, washed the swelling with it, and laid down to sleep. I slept for four hours, and on rising did not find a single sign of the swelling on my fingers or arm. The recoveries from rattlesnake bites under its action are affected in from two to twelve hours" (King 1887, p. 210).

A letter to the editor of the Lloyd Brothers' periodical, *The Gleaner,* reported on an Eclectic physician's use of Echinacea for venomous snake bites. "I have never found anything equal to Echinacea in treating blood poisoning or snake bite. I wish to report a case. A child was bitten on the big toe by a large rattlesnake. Forty-eight hours later the foot was greatly swollen and black as ink. The foot was bandaged with solutions of equal parts Specific Medicine Echinacea and water, and Echinacea was given internally, ten-drop doses every two hours. Complete recovery followed" (*The Gleaner* 1928b, p. 1079).

Dr. A. F. Stephens provided details on the treatment "for venomous bites and stings. Give 15–60 drops [tincture] in a little water every fifteen to thirty minutes. Keep bandage over affected area saturated, first full strength, afterward mixed with three parts water. Hypodermic indications about wound if necessary" (Stephens 1913, p. 133).

As early as 1915, Dr. Victor von Unruh of New York City made one of the earliest observations on the effects of Echinacea on white blood cells: "More than one hundred blood counts were made in cases of infectious diseases, mainly in tuberculosis. The results showed that Echinacea increases the phagocytic power of the leukocytes; it normalizes the percentage count of neutrophiles (Arneth count). Hyperleukocytosis and leukopenia are directly improved by Echinacea; the proportion of white to red blood cells is rendered normal; and the elimination of waste products is stimulated to a

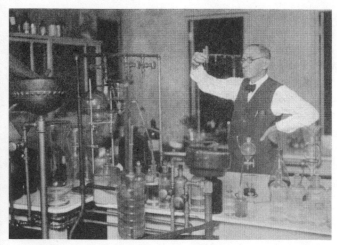

John Uri Lloyd in his laboratory

degree which puts this drug first rank among all alteratives" (Ellingwood 1915, p. 358).

Unruh went further in his observations and his praise: "Suffice it to say at this time that Echinacea does produce in the blood effects parallel with and similar to those produced by vaccines, without any of the objectionable features of the latter. The leucocytes are directly stimulated by Echinacea, their activity is increased, the percentage among the different classes of neutrophiles is rendered normal, and phagocytosis is thus raised to its best functioning capacity" (Unruh 1916, p. 64).

In the words of another Eclectic, A. M. Liebstein, "Nature has probably destined Echinacea to be used for remedial purposes only, as a sustainer of vitality, an organizer of the defensive powers of the system, to such an extant as to be justly crowned the greatest immunizing agent in the entire vegetable kingdom, as far as is known to medical science" (Liebstein 1927, pp. 316–17).

4
Modern Research and
Future Potential

Before the use of Echinacea in the United States fell into obscurity in the 1930s, the Eclectics had developed a fairly clear understanding of its mode of action.

It is not necessary to assume that a remedy must have a direct chemical effect upon bacteria for it to have germ-destroying action. The human body undoubtedly possesses the power to destroy such organisms, not only with the action of the blood corpuscles, but by means that we do not yet understand. A remedy may increase this germ resistance power, without in any way falling into the class of antiseptics. I do not mean to say that Echinacea has a direct anti-septic effect, but rather, that it has a revitalizing action upon those tissues that resist the action of pathogenic bacteria (*The Gleaner* 1928a, p. 1054).

When that anonymous writer wrote those words in 1928, little did he or she know that in fact later research would prove those words intuitive, timeless, and true. From 1940 through the present time, there have been over 200 papers published on the chemistry, pharmacology, and clinical applications of *E. purpurea,* and to a lesser extent *E. angustifolia* and *E. pallida.* German researchers have performed most of the studies, with results published in their language. A complete survey of the German studies is reviewed by Christopher Hobbs (1989) in his excellent work *The Echinacea Handbook.*

Echinacea became known in Europe around 1895, primarily for use in homeopathic practice. Interest in the plant grew to such proportions in Europe that severe shortages of supply were experienced. In 1937, for example, almost the entire crop was bought up by the French. German firms had difficulty obtaining limited amounts of the fresh plant. This prompted Dr. Gerhard Madaus of the firm Dr. Madaus & Co. (now of Cologne) to investigate cultivation of Echinacea in Europe. Dr. Madaus traveled to the United States in search of cuttings or seed. He was unable to obtain plant material from botanical gardens. He was able, however, to secure several ounces of *"E. angustifolia"* seed from Vaughn's Seed Store in Chicago. Dr. Madaus returned to Germany with the seed and established experimental plantings. The resulting plants turned out to be *E. purpurea* instead of *E. angustifolia.* Desiring fresh plant material for product manufacturing, the Madaus Company began a systematic investigation of the medicinal value of *E. purpurea,* which until that point, had only been mentioned in passing references in obscure and dated medical texts.   The result was that the vast majority of European pharmacological, clinical and chemical studies that have been conducted over the past fifty years have involved *E. purpurea,* primarily in the form of Echinacin®, a concentrate made from the fresh expressed juice of flowering *E. purpurea* manufactured by the Madaus firm (Hahn and Mayer, n.d.). Product forms include an ointment, liquid form for external use, an extract for internal use, as well as intravenous and intramuscular ampoules.

Important conclusions drawn from the research suggests Echinacea and its preparations are effective in treating certain viral infections, bacterial infections, healing wounds, and allaying inflammations, while stimulating the immune system. The most important of the dozens of pharmacological and clinical studies on Echinacea are reviewed below.

Pharmacological and Clinical Findings, 1939–1965

Early studies by Albus and Hering (1941), Fischer (1939), and Kriesbisch (1939) observed that various diseases caused by microorganisms responded favorably to local or intravenous therapy with Echinacea preparations despite the fact that Echinacea did not have a direct action against the disease-causing pathogens. Albus and Hering noted that the constituents of *E. purpurea* seemed to activate tissue functions that are in some way connected with the body's own healing powers.

Studies by E. Koch (1940), Albus and Hering (1941), and Geisbert (1943) also provided evidence that when applied locally to secondary skin infections or chronic suppurative wounds, that there was a proliferative tissue reaction that stimulated the development of granulation and healthy cells. Haase (1943), Philippart (1944), and Wember (1953) reported on the utility of Echinacea products in inflammatory conditions of the ear, nose, and throat. The utility of Echinacea in chronic pelvic inflammatory diseases was reported by Moell (1951a, 1951b) and Röseler (1952). The use of Echinacea in the treatment of inflammatory conditions of the prostate, urethra, and epididymis (a small organ attached to the testicles) was reported by H. A. Siggelkow (1942), C. E. Alken (1951), G. Herrmann (1952), and K. M. Bauer (1957, 1958). These early reports set the stage for future pharmacological studies that began to unlock the pharmacological action of Echinacea.

A 1950 study by Stoll, Renz, and Brack at Sandoz Co. isolated two glycosides from Echinacea exhibiting mild antibiotic activity against streptococci and *Staphylococcus aureus.* The most active of the two was a water-soluble crystalline compound, echinacoside, comprising one percent of the root preparation. It was then thought to be found only in *E. angustifolia,* but has since been found to be common to most species of Echinacea (Bauer and Foster 1989).

K. H. Büsing (1952, 1955) of the Hygiene Institute of the University of Marburg, in a search for the mechanism for Echinacea's action, began studying the effect of Echinacin® on the enzyme system called hyaluronidase. Hylauronidase regulates the polymerization, hence viscosity of cement substances in cellular connective tissue, such as hyaluronic acid. Hyaluronic acid is a mucopolysaccharide which is found in the ground substance of connective tissue.

The ground substance is the material that occupies spaces between cells and connective tissue. Hyaluronic acid acts both as a binding and protective agent. According to Büsing, the state of viscosity of the cement substances between the cells is important for adhering to or trapping microorganisms that enter tissue. Hyaluronidase regulates the polymerization of hyaluronic acid, and during the infection process can cause the breakdown of hyaluronic acid. Hyaluronic acid regulates the exchange of fluid and metabolites between cells, as well as vessel walls and cells. The greater resistance (higher viscosity), the better the chances of hyaluronic acid protecting against the spread of an infection.

He notes that a number of types of bacteria produce their own hyaluronidase, which can break down hyaluronic acid in mammals. Under certain environmental conditions, pathogenic bacteria (including streptococci, staphylococci, and pneumonococci) form "capsules" using hyaluronic acid, then utilize hyaluronidase as a pathway to enter tissue of the body. Therefore, Büsing set out to investigate whether extracts of the fresh expressed juice of *E. purpurea* could somehow inhibit depolymerized hyaluronidase, or conversely whether they could help to stabilize hyaluronic acid. His results showed that the Echinacea extracts helped to raise tissue resistance against pathogens by stabilizing hyaluronic acid and inactivating hyaluronidase produced by the bacteria, as well as that intrinsic to animal cellular tissue. At the same time the hyaluronidase-based intercellular cement retained a state of high polymerization, which provided effective resistance to the spread of bacteria. Büsing states that these pharmacological mechanisms provide an explanation for the efficacy of Echinacin®, at least for local applications, in infections of varied origin.

In 1952 Dr. E. Koch and H. Hasse of the biological institute of the Madaus company in Cologne also published their findings on the effect of Echinacin® on the hyaluronic acid/hyaluronidase system. The study was called "a modification of the spreading test in experimental animals: a contribution to the mechanism of action of Echinacin®." They found that 0.04 ccm of a fresh plant extract of *E. purpurea,* injected together with animal hyaluronidase, produced a strong hyaluronidase-inhibitory action corresponding to 1 mg of cortisone. Higher concentrations of the *Echinacea* extract (7:1) completely inhibited hyaluronidase.

A 1953 study, "Echinacin® and phagocyte reaction," conducted by O. Kuhn at the Zoological Institute of the University of Cologne found that substances present in Echinacin® (which at that time were still unidentified) had a number of pharmacological mechanisms. Confirming earlier studies, he again showed that the unknown substances in the plant inhibited hyaluronidase produced in the body, as well as that produced by microorganisms. Echinacea activates fibroblasts (cells that develop connective tissue), transforming them into cells that in turn produce hyaluronic acid. Echinacea activates phagocytic (particle-ingesting) white blood cells, as well as histiocytes (connective tissue cells with the ability for ameboid movement and phagocytic activity). The Echinacea components stimulate the regeneration of the cellular connective tissue and epidermal cells. In his paper, Kuhn reviewed previous studies and performed further research to interpret the data from a standpoint of developmental physiology. Results showed that Echinacin® activates phagocytosis by granulocytes. He found that experimental infections caused by streptococci in the blood would encounter two possibilities in contact with tissue pretreated with Echinacin®. Either an infective lesion failed to develop or the defensive mechanisms of the body were stimulated to prevent any spread of an infection, eliminating it in a few days.

E. Koch and H. Uebel (1953a) of the biological institute of the Madaus company found that guinea pigs treated with subcutaneous injections of Echinacea and then subjected to streptococci infections, exhibited a marked inhibition of bacterial cell growth compared to control animals. The effects of Echinacin® were again attributed to its ability to inhibit hyaluronidase while stimulating the regeneration of cellular connective tissue.

Koch and Uebel (1953b) also performed a study to determine the influence of *E. purpurea* on the hypophysis adrenals. This study involved intravenous applications of Echinacin® in guinea pigs that resulted in an increase of plasmalogen and cholesterol esters, and a fall of ascorbic acid. In the animal experiments, they showed that Echinacin® induced histological, chemical, and anatomical changes in the adrenal cortex. The kind of changes reported are associated with an increase in adrenocortical activity. Statistically significant increases in mitosis (cell division) and a rise in adrenal weights were also observed. The study showed that large doses of Echinacin® do not cause destructive changes in the adrenals or other toxic side effects.

Another Koch and Uebel (1954) study on the local influence of cortisone and Echinacin® on tissue resistance against streptococcus infection found that after pretreatment of guinea pigs with cortisone, the infection spread rapidly in the area. Pretreatment with Echinacin® resulted in the localization of the infection. Cortisone applications after previous infections also resulted in the spreading of the area and depth of the infection, whereas treatment with Echinacin® limited it to the original area of infection.

A study by a Russian researcher, B.S. Nikol'sakaya (1954), that tested blood-clotting and wound-healing properties of various plant preparations in rabbit blood—including a preparation of *E. purpurea*—found that in doses of 2 ml/kg, blood clotting was increased thirty minutes after administration and hastened the wound-healing process. Of the other plants tested, *Plantago psyllium* (pysllium) had no blood-clotting effect, but hastened healing; *Pulmonaria officinalis* (lungwort) and *Senecio fuchsii* exhibited no wound-healing or blood-clotting effects; and *Plantago major* (common plantain) showed marked wound-healing activity, but no blood-clotting effects.

Researchers F. K. Tünnerhoff and H. K. Schwabe (1956) of the Medical Clinic of the University of Bonn undertook a number of studies on the effect of Echinacea concentrate on artificial connective tissue formation after fibrin implantation in both animals and humans. In the healing process fibrin is transformed (by amino acids) to provide raw material used by the body in the development of connective tissue ground substance. In this series of experiments, the researchers found that Echinacin®-fibrin implants increased the rate of healing and produced young fibroblasts more rapidly compared with pure fibrin implants. This difference in the formation of tissue was in part attributed to the antihyaluronidase activity of Echinacin®. They further surmised that Echinacin® exerts a protective action on intercellular polysaccharides produced by fibrocytes (inactive cells produced by fibroblasts). They found large amounts of the polysaccharides in the Echinacin®-fibrin grafts, but only small amounts in the pure fibrin grafts. Echinacin® stimulated young fibroblasts to transform mucopolysaccharides into connective tissue. As did Koch and Haase (1952), Tünnerhoff and Schwabe concluded that Echinacin® reduced vascular permeability within a wound and hindered diffusion.

K. H. Büsing (1958) performed a study on the effect of a preparation from the fresh expressed juice of *E. purpurea* (Echinacin®) on properdin levels in rabbits. Properdin is a serum protein that in the presence of magnesium ions and a chemical complement has the capability to help neutralize viruses and bacteria (Taber 1970). Properdin, acting in conjunction with a chemical complement, binds to bacteria and viral polysaccharides with high affinity, rendering them harmless. This study showed that intravenous injections of Echinacea extract at 0.6 ml/kg initially decreased properdin levels. After about twenty hours, however, such injections strongly increased the levels to the point where they remained far above normal for at least 120 hours. Büsing and Thüringen (1958) reported similar results in which intravenous injections of *E. purpurea* extracts in rabbits at first produced a lowering in serum properdin, followed by a significant reactive increase of properdin levels (50 to 70 percent).

A. Mostbeck and M. Studlar (1962) of Vienna reported on an experimental investigation of a plant extract from *E. purpurea* (Echinacin®) as a nonspecific immunostimulant, with special reference to its influence on the adrenal cortex. The adrenal cortex system secretes a large number of substances, including over forty steroids that affect and regulate the metabolism of proteins and carbohydrates, water and electrolyte metabolism, and sex hormones. This clinical study involved thirty-one patients. After intravenous injection of one or two ampules of an injectable form of Echinacin®, eosinophil leucocyte counts were reduced by 50 percent in twenty-five out of thirty-one subjects. Following the animal studies by Koch and Uebel (1953b), Mostbeck and Studlar also performed an experiment to determine the level of steroid excretions in the urine of nineteen subjects, twelve hours after the administration of one ampoule of intravenous Echinacin®. The rise in steroid excretion averaged 146 percent. The vast majority of subjects also experienced a raise in temperature within three hours after receiving the injection. They concluded that one of the principal effects of the intravenous injections appeared to be the stimulation of hormone production in the adrenal cortex system, which serves to support previous clinical usage in the use of the Echinacea injection for chronic inflammatory conditions.

G. Orzechowski (1963) performed histological studies that showed that Echinacin® was able to speed up the differentiation of fibroblasts and fibrocytes.

A 1965 study by B. Chone demonstrated that, after rabbits were injected with a polysaccharide fraction from *E. purpurea,* the number of circulating granulocytes increased.

Antiviral Research

When cells are exposed to viruses, interferon (one or more proteins that help to protect noninfected cells against viral infections), is formed. In a 1976 dissertation produced by H. G. Eilmes at the University of Frankfurt, the author provided evidence for interferon-like activity in relation to the glycoside echinacoside (isolated as a pure compound) as well as a whole plant extract of Echinacea. The whole extract had greater activity than the pure chemical compound, suggesting that chemical components other than echinacoside were involved in the interferonlike activity.

A 1978 study by A. Wacker and A. Hilbig of the Center for Biological Chemistry of the University of Frankfurt found that Echinacin® possessed an interferon like activity in protecting cells against viral-induced canker sores (vesicular stomatitis), influenza, and herpes. They found that *E. purpurea* only had an antiviral effect if mammalian cells were pretreated with Echinacea. This rendered the cells virus-resistant. Once preincubated in this way, there was no longer any need for the addition of more Echinacea. The authors noted that it was in this way that the action of Echinacea resembles the mode of action of interferon. Fractionated components were tested to determine if the antiviral activity could be found in a single chemical fraction, but they found that the antiviral activity was spread over several chemical fractions.

The research team of D. Orinda, J. Diederich, and A. Wacker (1973) had published previously on the antiviral activity of *E. purpurea*. Using this work and experience gained in interferon research, they showed that interferon-induced substances such as Echinacea did not have to come into contact with viruses to inhibit them. Rather, they found that mammalian cells had to be pretreated with the virus-inhibiting substance. Cells so treated achieve viral resistance for a certain period of time, then become susceptible once again. In the present study they found that mammalian cells had to be pretreated four to six hours before the virus attack, and that this protection lasted for a period of twenty-four to forty-eight hours.

Another 1978 study by May and Willuhn reported on a screening test of water extracts of various plants for antiviral activity against herpes, influenza, vaccinia, and polio virus. Root extracts of *E. angustifolia* produced no effects in the assay system. However, one must question the identity of the *E. angustifolia* in this study in light of the misidentification problems persistent between *E. angustifolia* and *E. pallida* that have recently come to light. On the other hand, *E. purpurea* inhibited the herpes and influenza viruses without demonstrating toxicity.

Studies on an Echinacea Combination

Th. Vömel of the University of Erlangen-Nürnberg reported in 1978 on the results of findings on the influence of immune system stimulators on the phagocytosis of erythrocytes (red blood corpuscles) by the reticulohistiocytary system of isolated perfused rat liver. Red blood cells have a life history estimated at an average of 120 days. Once they die and disintegrate, the debris is phagocytosed (ingested) by cells of the reticuloendothelial system (RES). Cells involved in the RES include macrophages and other groups of cells in the body with ability to ingest foreign or worn-out cells or substances, including worn-out red blood cells. Cells of the RES are involved in helping repair injured tissue and in cell-mediated immune defense mechanisms. Some of the debris produced by disintegrating red blood cells, including proteins and iron, are stored by the RES cells, then recirculated back into the formation of new red blood cells. When the body is in balance, this complex system is remarkably efficient.

In Vömel's experiment, a commercial product named Esberitox®, containing fresh leaf extracts of *Thuja occidentalis* (White Cedar), root tincture of *Baptisia tinctoria* (Wild Indigo), and root extracts of *E. angustifolia* and *E. purpurea*, was tested along with single extracts of the plant materials. The phagocytosis of erythrocytes was significantly improved by both the combination and the single extracts. The *Thuja occidentalis* extract showed the greatest effect on the first phase of phagocytosis. Single extracts of *E. purpurea* showed the most influence over phagocytosis-dependent metabolism.

A number of other studies have been published on the clinical applications of Esberitox®. Since this product contains other plant materials in addition to Echinacea, it is difficult to extrapolate the results of those studies to Echinacea preparations. However, some studies have compared Esberitox® with Echinacea extracts. Helbig (1961) reported on results of a controlled comparative study on the use of this Esberitox® as a preventative and therapeutic agent in upper respiratory tract infections of 644 children. Kleinschmidt (1965), also in a controlled comparative study, tested the effects of the preparation in influenza in 209 children. Compared with the control group, there was a significant reduction in the rate of infection. In a year-long controlled comparative study involving 286 children in a

German children's home, Freyer (1974) showed that Esberitox® had a preventive action on colds and influenza, significantly reducing the rate of infection.

A number of studies reported on the effects of the Echinacea combination in radiology patients. P. Pohl (1969) demonstrated that treatment with Esberitox® preparations in radiology patients resulted in the enhancement of leukocyte production in the bone marrow. The average period of administration (24.4 days) produced an average increase of 15.5 percent in leukocytes. Similar results were obtained in a study by Sartor (1972). Kärcher used Esberitox® in the Radiation Treatment Clinic in Vienna and found that the preparation was of value in determining bone marrow reserves in radiology patients who developed leukopenia (abnormal decrease in white blood cell production, which is often a side effect of radiation therapy).

B. Chone and B. Manidakis (1969) and Manidakis (1968) used Echinacin® to develop the leukocyte provocation test. Since Echinacin® intravenous injections cause a rise in body temperature and an increase in the leukocyte count, this property of Echinacin® was used to develop the diagnostic test. Before and after extensive supervolt therapy, the test was performed in fifty-three patients. It proved useful as an estimate of bonemarrow reserve. After the administration of Echinacin® a low leukocyte count was used to indicate impairment of the bone marrow reserve. The described test is considered simple, without risk, and usually obviates the need for further diagnostic tests. Lorenz and Messner (1974) and Lorenz *et al.* (1972) used a similar method to diagnose bone marrow function in children with viral hepatitis. During the course of viral hepatitis, the test was able to show the incidence of reversible bone marrow depression.

S. A. Qadripur (1976) investigated the effects of Esberitox® on bacterial infections in patients at the Dermatological Hospital in Göttingen. Qadripur showed that bacterial skin infections in humans could be healed completely and rapidly as the result of an improvement in the phagocytosis rate. Patients involved in this double-blind study had bacterial skin infections and exhibited limited phagocytosis function.

The Use of Echinacea for Skin Diseases and Wounds

A number of reports have confirmed the value of Echinacin® as a therapeutic agent both in activating defenses and the redevelopment of tissue in inflamed skin injuries. Topical products have been used clinically since the 1940s. Injectable or oral forms of Echinacea have also been used alongside more accepted forms of treatment for skin conditions such as psoriasis and eczema.

F. Schnurbusch (1955) published on the utility of Echinacea in the treatment of the skin condition pemphigus vulgaris. Korting and Born (1954) and Korting and Rasp (1954) reported on the utility of Echinacea as an adjunct therapy in treating psoriasis. In the later report, Echinacin® injections were used as an adjunct treatment in twenty-nine psoriasis patients who were also treated with conventional topical treatments. The Echinacea injections reduced relapse tendencies of the condition. Using oral dosages of Echinacin®, W. Gaertner (1963) found that in conjunction with conventional topical therapies, 90 percent of the 200 patients studied had definite remissions in psoriasis. The treatment was continued over a long period, from nine to eighteen months. In 1967 H. Tronnier reported on the successful use of Echinacin® injections as an immune system stimulant for certain forms of eczema, particular chronic or recurrent cases.

Recent pharmacological and clinical studies provide evidence for the mode of action of topical products and their therapeutic potential in clinical practice.

In a study involving 109 patients with burns, minor skin injuries, and leg ulcers, Mund-Hoym (1979) confirmed anti-inflammatory and healing-promoting effects of external use of the preparation. Mund-Hoym reported that one of the most impressive examples of efficacy was the ability of the Echinacea preparations to rapidly cleanse wound surfaces of dirt particles, especially in sports-related abrasions. Complete healing without complications was achieved in 87 percent of cases. First-degree burns were reported to heal promptly. Additional medications or therapeutic procedures were used in the management of second- and third-degree burns, followed by external application of Echinacea. Again the results were positive. Positive surface reactions in the application of Echinacea external products to minor injuries was achieved in three to four days in twenty-two out of twenty-six patients observed.

An early study by Viehmann (1978) described the therapeutic success of Echinacin® ointment with a success rate of 85.5 percent in 4598 (2421 men and 2164 women) patients with similar skin injuries as described above. The ointment contains 16.0 g per 100 g of the juice extracted from the fresh, flowering, above-ground parts of *E. purpurea*. The study lasted for about five months and involved the observations of 538 physicians (outside of hospitals) from all parts of West Germany. Skin conditions were divided into six different categories: Predominantly inflammatory skin conditions involved 212 patients, with a success rate of 85.4 percent in 8.5 days recorded. The wound category recorded the physicians' experience with 1453 patients, with successful healing recorded in 91.5 percent of cases. Eczema cases included 628 patients, with a 82.3 percent success rate of treatment. Burns involved 626 patients, with a 96.3 percent healing rate recorded. The fifth category, herpes simplex, achieved a success rate of 91.4 percent in 222 cases. In 900 cases of varicose ulcers, beneficial results were achieved in 71.1 percent of cases. The author of the study concluded that the *E. purpurea* ointment was a highly effective topical agent for several types of skin lesions, including all types of wounds, burns, eczema, inflammatory skin conditions, herpes simplex, and varicose ulcers of the leg. Side effects were reported in 2.3 percent of patients and included "burning pain" and intensified itching. Such cases were recorded as intolerance to the ointment.

While this type of study does not possess the statistical status of a controlled trial, a large number of doctors and patients were involved. Double-blind or single-blind clinical trials for the conditions treated are considered difficult to perform in general medical practice, and raise ethical questions as well.

These and other studies on topical application of Echinacea products have shown a general beneficial influence on chronic suppurative wounds, eczema eruptions, and eruptions of secondarily infected skin, as well as general infections where healing is dependent upon the formation of granulation tissue and relatively rapid healing of tissue cells. In reviewing the therapeutic efficacy of Echinacin® ointment in general practice for skin lesions, K. Sickel (1971), a general practitioner in Cologne, lists the action of the ointment as involving rapid wound cleansing, elimination of dirt particles, avoidance of secondary infections, avoidance of wound complications, relief of pain, a sensation of coolness, plus rapid formation of granulation tissue, formation of skin epidermis, and a general avoidance of scars.

A 1984 study by H. J. Kinkel, M. Plate, and H.-U. Tüllner of Dr. Madaus & Co. reported on the effect of Echinacin® ointment in the healing of skin lesions. This animal study was performed to develop comparative, reproducible models of evaluation for further understanding of the clinical picture of wounds, and to help quantify the action of Echinacea ointment on the healing process of wounds. Guinea pigs with skin wounds were treated with the ointment. On the sixth and ninth days after treatment, the lesion area was significantly smaller in those treated with the salve compared with controls. A significant improvement was observed after three days.

In 1987 F. K. Meißner published on his findings on experimental studies of the mode of action of Echinacin® on skin flap necrosis. The rate of necrosis of skin flaps in animal experiments was studied comparing the Echinacea preparation to NaCl and pentoxifylline. The noncirculated area of the skin flap was significantly smaller in Echinacea-treated animals than in controls. The Echinacea preparation proved to produce a significant decrease of the rate of necrosis of skin flaps in test animals.

Researchers A. Tubaro *et. al.*, from institutions in Trieste and Milan, Italy, reported in a 1987 study on the "anti-inflammatory activity of a polysaccharide fraction of *E. angustifolia.*" Polysaccharide fractions of *E. angustifolia* roots were tested on carrageenan-induced paw edema and croton oil-induced ear edema of mice. The paw edema was almost completely inhibited over an eight-hour period, and applied topically, reduced the ear edema as well. The fraction also reduced leukocytic infiltration of the croton oil dermatitis. The fractions appeared slightly less effective as an anti-inflammatory agent than indomethacin. The conclusion was that anti-inflammatory activity of Echinacea appeared, at least in part, to be the result of the polysaccharide content.

The Use of Echinacea in the Treatment of Lung Conditions

D. Baetgen (1964) and O. Zimmerman (1969) reported that intramuscular injections of Echinacin® (1–2 ml.), given consecutively over three days, could reduce the severity and duration of paroxysms in whooping cough, while shortening the convulsive stage of the disease. Baetgen's study involved 121 children. About half of the patients were free of symptoms within five days, while the other half recovered in ten days. Zimmerman's study included 91 patients. The length of the illness was shortened, and no side effects were attributed to Echinacin®.

O. Sprockhoff (1964) reported on positive results in the use of Echinacin® injections for the treatment of a number of conditions in clinical pediatric practice, including pertussis and bronchitis (with spasms), inflammatory bone conditions, and tonsillitis.

W. Heesen (1964) reported on the use of Echinacin® as an adjunct therapy to raise immune system resistance in infections with *Mycrobacterium tuberculosis*. Improvement was noted in the treatment of several hundred patients, especially those resistant to conventional therapies or those with progressive tuberculosis.

In a 1978 review article on the diagnosis and treatment of upper respiratory tract infections, K. D. Tympner suggested Echinacea injections should be used as a way to increase resistance to infections in children.

An injectable form of Echinacin® was used in a 1984 study by D. Baetgen to test the effect of the drug in the treatment of pertussis in children. Three doses of an injection of 2 ml per day was given over three consecutive days to children, and 1 ml per day to infants. In one third of the cases the duration of pertussis was reduced to five days. The treatment was particularly successful at early stages of the condition. Combinations of the injection with antibiotics were also used, but were not equally effective. However, the author concluded that the combined treatment may be more effective than antibiotic treatment alone.

Baetgen (1988) published results obtained in a retrospective comparative study on the use of Echinacin® injections in the treatment of viral infections of the respiratory tract in 1280 young children. The injections were given in a course of three to four injections on consecutive days. The study showed that the treatment can significantly shorten the duration of the infections compared with other treatment methods. Baetgen reported notable improvement in patients diagnosed with "dry cough involving the lungs" or "obstructive bronchitis." If antibiotics were given in conjunction with the Echinacin® injections, the improvement took significantly longer.

Allergies

A 1978 study by German researcher Franz Josef Reith showed that capsules and tablets containing whole plants or plant parts of *E. purpurea* and *E. angustifolia,* plus lactic acid, were effective in the treatment of numerous allergies.

Studies on the Use of Echinacea for *Candida* Infections

E. Coeugniet and R. Kühnast published their findings in a 1986 paper on the effects of Echinacin® as an immunostimulating agent against candidal mycosis. Econazole nitrate cream, an antifungal agent, was applied locally for about six days in all cases. Both injectable and oral forms of the Echinacea extract were used to enhance nonspecific, cell-mediated immunity. The frequency of recurrence with those treated only with econazole nitrate was 60.5 percent. This rate was improved by 5 percent and 16 percent (depending upon the form of application) in patients treated with the Echinacea preparations. During the trial, 203 patients diagnosed with recurrent candidal inflammation of the vagina and/or vulvitis were treated between 1983 and 1985. Further results on the use of Echinacea in the treatment of candida infections were reported by Coeugniet (1988).

J.R. Möse (1983) of the Institute of Hygiene, University of Graz, reported on the results of a study on the effect of Echinacin® on phagocytic activity and natural killer cells. Twelve healthy male subjects were studied to ascertain the phagocytic activity against *Candida albicans,* and how leukocytes behaved in a natural killer cell test (with K 562 cells), before, during, and after administration of the Echinacea preparation. Statistical analysis of test results showed that Echinacin® produced a marked increase in phagocytic efficiency. The effect lasted up to the end of the experiment following a four-day period of administration. The behavior of natural killer cells under the influence of Echinacea did not result in any definite conclusions.

Clinical Experience in Rheumatoid Arthritis

A number of early papers by H. K. L. Meißner (1950a, 1950b, 1951, 1953), A. Schuster (1952), and M. Broglie (1954) reported on the use of Echinacin® in the treatment of rheumatoid arthritis. Based on his clinical experience in the use of intravenous injections of Echinacin® in the treatment of chronic polyarthritis, D. Reuß, a general practitioner from Kuchen, West Germany, published the results of his work in 1986 (see also D. Reuß 1979, 1981). The disease, variously termed progressive polyarthritis, rheumatoid arthritis, or chronic primary polyarthritis, poses problems for physicians in general practice. Reuß did not obtain what he considered to be satisfactory results with better-known drugs (cortisone, gold, and penicillamine) for the symptomatic treatment of the condition. In his search for alternative therapies, he used Echinacin® injections. While he admits his case histories do not hold the statistical weight of double-blind studies, he notes that the positive results he has obtained in over thirty years experience in treating patients with Echinacin® (in the early stages of chronic polyarthritis) warrants the development of future double-blind trials. While the treatment did not produce results in advanced cases of the disease, in early stages Reuß noted marked improvement ranging from relief of pain in the finger joints to freedom from symptoms, which he says could be expected with reasonable certainty in almost every case. He expressed regrets that this simple and uncomplicated form of treatment for such a problematic disease had not reached a place in official medicine, and hoped that his experience would stimulate further research, free from prejudice.

In Search of Immunostimulants

Immunostimulants are agents that stimulate the immune system in a nonspecific manner. The pharmacological effects of nonspecific immunostimulants fade relatively quickly, and have to be administered quite frequently or continuously. An increase in phagocytosis (by macrophages) and granulocytes are important factors in immunostimulation. Immunostimulants could become alternative or adjuncts to chemotherapy, and may help prevent infections by activating the immune system in persons whose immune response has become impaired. This is in no way to imply that the use of Echinacea could in any way be useful to HIV-infected individuals. Immunostimulants are potentially useful in some cancers and infectious disease (Wagner and Proksch 1985). The immune system-related research on Echinacea over the last decade is an important scientific development in Echinacea research. The research group headed by H. Wagner at the Institute of Pharmaceutical Biology, University of Munich, has published a number of reviews on fungi and flowering plants with immunostimulant potential (Wagner 1981, Wagner 1984, Wagner 1986a, Wagner 1986b, Wagner and Proksch 1985, and Wagner *et al.* 1985).

Intensive research on the use of Echinacea as a nonspecific immune system stimulant evolved considerably in the 1970s. Research conducted by Italian researchers I. Bonadeo, G. Botazzi, and M. Lavazza (1971) revealed further mechanisms for Echinacea's wound-healing capacity. They isolated a polysaccharide named "echinacin B" from *E. angustifolia*. Polysaccharides are complex carbohydrates, usually of high molecular weight, that can be broken down into two or more simple sugars. The Italian researchers theorized that echinacin B (polysaccharide) formed a complex with hyaluronic acid that resulted in the inhibition of depolymerization of hyaluronic acid by hyaluronidase. Other pharmacological mechanisms observed included the organization of the fibrous insoluble protein found in connective tissue (collagen), increasing viscosity of tissue ground substance, and a reaction resulting in the proliferation of fibroblasts (connective tissue-forming cells). The stabilization and temporary increase of hyaluronic acid by the effect of echinacin B, coupled with the increase of connective tissue-forming cells (fibroblasts), forms the basis of the wound-healing process.

In 1981 researchers H. Wagner and A. Proksch of the Institute of Pharmaceutical Biology, University of Munich, published their finding on the discovery of two polysaccharides in *E. purpurea* that stimulated T-cell activity 20 to 30 percent more than a highly potent T-cell stimulator. T-cells are a type of white blood cell (leukocytes) categorized as lymphocytes. They are produced in the bone marrow, thymus gland, and other lymphoid tissues. They are stored in the lymph nodes and spleen. They travel to the site of infections, combine with antigens, and release various chemicals that are in part responsible for cell-mediated immunity.

In this important study, Wagner and Proksch (1981a) demonstrated in various test systems that the polysaccharides produced a maximum increase in phagocytosis in the carbon clearance test and T-lymphocyte transformation test. The carbon clearance test measures the rate of elimination of carbon particles from the blood when injected into the peritoneum. The rate of elimination indicates the efficiency or phagocytosis activity of the phagocytic system (Wagner

1986a). Phagocytosis is a major factor in nonspecific immune defense. The test reveals information on the activity and function of phagocytes. Wagner and Proksch also measured the effect of the polysaccharides in the T-lymphocyte transformation test. This test measures the multiplication (by budding) of normal lymphocytes after contact with a substance that causes cell division. The resulting rate of cell division is then measured. Other tests were used to explore the polysaccharide's spectrum of activity, all of which produced positive results. Wagner and Proksch (1981b) were able to isolate and identify two polysaccharides, deemed polysaccharide I and polysaccharide II.

"Changes to the immunological parameters in people by *E. purpurea*" is a 1986 study by M. Gaisbauer and W. Zimmerman of the Hospital for Natural Healing, Munich, and T. Schleich of the Technological University, Munich. The study focused on the effects of an aqueous extract of *E. purpurea* and an "Echinacea complex" on helper and suppressor cytotoxic lymphocytes subjected to snake and bee poisons. In both cases, a significant increase in the total number of lymphocytes was observed. Similar results were obtained in an 1987 study by Gaisbauer *et al.*

In 1986 H. Enbergs and A. Woestmann of the University of Bonn published findings on a study on "The effects of *E. angustifolia* on phagocytic activity of peripheral leukocytes of rabbits." Extracts were administered at various dilutions in a 1 ml. subcutaneous dose. No treatment or placebo groups were used as controls. An analytical method (chemoluminescence) of whole blood samples was used to determine the phagocytic activity of peripheral leukocytes. The study included four separate experiments over five and six days. The total leukocyte count in peripheral blood of all animals was in the normal range, and *E. angustifolia* produced no effects using this parameter. However, the authors concluded *E. angustifolia* preparations resulted in an increase in phagocytic activity. Half-strength and undiluted *E. angustifolia* preparations produced statistically significant results.

A 1987 study conducted by Angelika Proksch and Hildebert Wagner of the Institute for Pharmaceutical Biology, University of

Munich, reported on the structure analysis of a 4-*O*-methyl-glucuronoarabinoxylan polysaccharide from *E. purpurea* with immunostimulating activity. The first report of a polysaccharide from *E. purpurea* with activity against hyaluronidase was reported, but without characterization, by Bonadeo *et al.* in 1971. Researchers at the University of Munich previously published on immunostimulant activity from polysaccharide fractions *in vitro* (in the laboratory) and *in vivo* (in living organisms) in 1981, 1984, and 1985. The 1987 study reported on the structure analysis of one of the isolated pure polysaccharides. The authors report that the heteroxylan of *E. purpurea* described in this article is one of the first polysaccharides in the Asteraceae (aster family) to be isolated in pure form with elucidation of its basic chemical structure. They further showed *in vitro* immunostimulating activity with the pure isolated compound. Previous studies had been on extracts of various plant parts or component groups, rather than pure, isolated polysaccharides.

Coeugniet and Elek (1987) studied commercial extracts of *Viscum album* (mistletoe) and *E. purpurea* to report the effects of the extracts on the production of lymphokines by lymphocytes and in a test known as the transformation test. They showed that clinical applications of the extracts produced stimulation of cell-mediated immunity after one therapeutic administration, followed by a week free from treatment. Conversely, they produced an immune depressive effect if high daily doses were given. However, these were clinically irrelevant, extremely high dosages.

H. Wagner, H. Stuppner, W. Schäfer, and M. Zenk published a 1988 study on the isolation of three polysaccharides from *E. purpurea* cell cultures. The paper described the isolation and structure determination of three polysaccharides from tissue culture that proved to be immunologically active. A fucogalactoxyloglucan was shown to enhance phagocytosis *in vitro* and *in vivo*. An arabinogalactan specifically stimulated macrophages to excrete the tumor necrosis factor. While similar, the polysaccharides obtained in tissue culture were not identical to polysaccharides extracted from the plant.

A study entitled "Immunological in vivo and in vitro examinations of extracts of the roots of *E. angustifolia, E. pallida,* and *E. purpurea* " by R. Bauer, K. Jurcic, H. Puhlmann, and H. Wagner (1988) examined the extracts in the carbon clearance test (carbon elimination) with mice and in the granulocyte test. Oral administration of all extracts was found to significantly enhance phagocytosis. In the carbon clearance test, *E. purpurea* produced a triple rate of elimination, while *E. angustifolia* and *E. pallida* exhibited double the rate of elimination compared with controls. The stimulation of phagocytosis in this *in vivo* test correlated with the *in vitro* granulocyte test. The authors reported that lipophilic (fat soluble) fractions of the extract appeared to more active than polar fractions. The researchers analyzed all extracts using HPLC (high pressure liquid chromatography) to correlate chemical constituents with immunological activities.

This study has a number of important implications for future directions in Echinacea research. The lipophilic fractions of extracts of these three species were without exception of stronger action than the hydrophilic (water soluble) fractions. Only in hydrophilic fractions of *E. purpurea* were positive immunological effects also noted. This study shows that the main active group of compounds is probably the isobutylamides and/or poline/enes of the essential oils (found in the lipophilic fractions). In the hydrophilic fractions of *E. purpurea,* caffeic acid derivatives are believed responsible for immunostimulation.

It has been previously stated in many reports, primarily anecdotally, that roots producing a tingling sensation on the tongue have the most therapeutic value. This tingling sensation is believed to be produced by the compounds in the isobutylamide group. Here it is shown for the first time that the lipophilic fractions of the roots of *E. angustifolia, E. pallida,* and *E. purpurea* had an immunological effect on the mononuclear phagocytic system. The presence of a tingling sensation on the tongue produced by an Echinacea species could serve as a primitive type of taste-test assay of quality.

Echinacoside, a phenol glycoside, was once believed primarily responsible for the biological activity of Echinacea. It was once known only from *E. angustifolia* and its presence had been used as a way to chemically distinguish that species from *E. purpurea,* which does not contain the component. However, Bauer, Khan, and Wagner (1988) found echinacoside in *E. pallida.* Bauer and Foster (1989) also reported on the occurrence of echinacoside in *E. simulata* and *E. paradoxa.* Echinacoside now seems to occur frequently in most species of Echinacea, though in a recent study, it was found to be surprisingly absent from *E. tennesseensis* (Bauer, Remiger, and Alstat 1990). Echinacoside has previously been shown to have weak bacteriostatic activity (Stoll, Renz, and Brack 1950). Bauer and his coworkers have concluded that echinacoside is probably not of importance as an active agent on the immune system.

Various studies, reported on above and below, support the claim that isolated polysaccharide fractions are immunologically active. However, in their study the authors note that the polysaccharides are probably not present in ethanol extracts (tinctures) of Echinacea because they precipitate in alcohol. Polysaccharides, however are found in some plant juice preparations or extracts with high water percentages. Therefore, the lipophilic fractions in commercial products, rather than polysaccharides, are probably of greater significance in immunostimulation in most high-ethanol commercial Echinacea preparations. R. Bauer, K. Jurcic, H. Puhlmann, and H. Wagner (1988) note, however, that a definitive coordination of compounds to specific immunological actions cannot be stated at this time. It is also impossible to answer the question, "which is the best Echinacea species," based on this study. While the majority of studies on immunological activity have been conducted with extracts of the expressed juice of *E. purpurea,* this study was also able to confirm immunological activity in the roots of *E. angustifolia* and *E. pallida.* Furthermore it justifies the interchangeable therapeutic use of these two species. Since the constituents of *E. pallida* are unstable in storage, the authors suggest, that it would be best to consider it a second official species next to *E. angustifolia.*

In 1988 Wagner, Stuppner, Schafer and Zenk isolated three

polysaccharides from cell cultures of *E. purpurea*, which were different in structure than the polysaccharide previously obtained by Proksch (1980). One of the polysaccharides obtained in cell culture (a fucogalactoxyloglucan of high molecular weight) enhanced phagocytosis in both *in vitro* and *in vivo* models. The third polysaccharide (an arabinogalactan) was shown to simulate macrophages to excrete the tumor necrosis factor. One way in which such laboratory research on pure compounds has practical value is when the substances can be reproduced in quantities large enough to be of possible economic value. A 1989 study by H. Wagner, H. Stuppner, J. Puhlmann, *et al.* produced tissue cultures of *E. purpurea* yielding two immunologically active polysaccharides (a neutral fucogalactoxyloglucan and an acidic arabinogalactan). The article reports on their isolation and elucidation, as well as the fact that they can be obtained in an industrial scale.

M. L. Lohmann-Matthes and H. Wagner (1989) published on research that showed polysaccharides from cell cultures of *E. purpurea* were found to be effective in activation of macrophages *in vitro* and *in vivo*. Macrophages were activated to cytotoxicity against tumor cells and microorganisms. Lethal infections of *Candida albicans* or *Listeria monocytogenes* in mice were efficiently managed by intravenous injections of the polysaccharides. The polysaccharides stimulated macrophages to produce tumor necrosis factor alpha, interleukin 1, and interferon beta.

As suggested by previous work of R. Bauer, a 1989 paper by R. Bauer, P. Remiger, K. Jurcic, and H. Wagner concluded that other constituents in addition to polysaccharides are responsible for phagocytosis-inducing activity in Echinacea. Ethanol extracts of both the roots and herb of *E. angustifolia, E. pallida,* and *E. purpurea* were found to influence phagocytosis *in vitro* and *in vivo.* Lipophilic constituents were shown to be the most active. Alkamide fractions also showed good activity and may have contributed to phagocytic stimulation of the alcohol extracts. Cichoric acid was also shown to produce stimulatory activity.

K. Jurcic, D. Melchart, M. Holzmann, P. Martin, R. Bauer, A. Doenecke, and H. Wagner reported on their findings in a 1989 paper on the influence of two preparations of Echinacea on the phagocytic activity of human granulocytes studied after intravenous and oral dosage in both single and double blind studies. Both of the preparations significantly enhanced phagocytic activity. The maximum phagocytic activity was attained in both studies after the fourth or fifth day of application.

Anticancer Potential?

A study conducted by USDA researchers Voaden and Jacobson in 1972 identified an oncolytic (destructive to tumors) hydrocarbon from the essential oils of *E. pallida* and *E. angustifolia*, and demonstrated that it possessed tumor-inhibiting capabilities. The component from the distilled oil from the roots was found to be active in inhibiting both Walker carcinosarcoma 256 and P-388 lymphocytic leukemia, though it was inactive in lymphoid leukemia.

These results (as in the results of all research) must be viewed in their intended context, and certainly should not be blown out of proportion. This study simply showed that a component identified from the essential oil had an adverse effect on certain forms of cancer cells in laboratory experiments. This type of screening is an initial research stage used to identify compounds (usually highly toxic) that might one day be used in chemotherapy. The assay used for Walker carcinosarcoma 256 has been abandoned because it was later found to be excessively sensitive, giving a large number of false positive leads (Cassady, Baird, and Chang 1990).

A research team headed by B. Leuttig of the Fraunhofer Institute for Toxicology and Immune Biology in Hannover, West Germany, along with scientists from the University of Munich and the University of Florida, Gainesville, reported on their findings on the activity of a polysaccharide from cell cultures of *E. purpurea*. The paper, published in the *Journal of the National Cancer Institute* (1989), reported on the effects of a highly purified polysaccharide (arabinogalactan), which the authors suggest may have implications in defense against tumors and infectious disease. They found that macrophages were activated to cytotoxicity against a line of tumor cells as well as a parasitic protozoan *Leishmania enriettii*. In a battery of laboratory tests they showed that the polysaccharide-induced macrophages to produce tumor necrosis factor, interleukin-1, and interferon-beta$_2$. The polysaccharide also produced a slight increase in T-cell proliferation. This research, using a highly purified chemical component from *E. purpurea* cell cultures, sets the stage for further work of a similar nature that could one day result in the development of a new drug for use against certain forms of cancer or infectious disease. It also helps scientists to understand the functions of activated macrophages in immune defense.

Conclusions

Over the past forty years, studies suggest and demonstrate that Echinacea is anti-inflammatory, has strong wound-healing action, stimulates the immune system, is effective against certain viral and bacterial infections, and is a potentially useful therapeutic agent in diseases from asthma to cancers.

Pharmacological research shows that Echinacea preparations help stimulate the body's own defense system of cellular immunity. Echinacea primarily works through stimulating cellular or nonspecific immunity, as opposed to specific immunity, such as that produced by antibodies reacting to a specific antigen (as in the way in which vaccines work). Echinacea seems to stimulate a complement of nonspecific mechanisms such as phagocytes and macrophages, which help to ingest and destroy invading particles. It stimulates the activity of leukocytes (various types of white blood corpuscles that act as scavengers in order to help combat infections). Components of Echinacea inhibit hyaluronidase, an enzyme involved in the infection process. Various components have mild bacteriostatic and fungistatic activity—helping to allay the spread of pathogens, rather than killing them outright, as an antibiotic would do. By increasing fibroblasts (cells involved in the development of connective tissue) it helps to stimulate new tissue development. Studies on properdin levels have shown that this serum protein complex—which helps activate various aspects of the immune system—is increased by Echinacea extracts, providing a further mechanism for its immunostimulatory action. Studies have also shown that Echinacea may also act through stimulating increased production of interferon by macrophages. In addition, Echinacea has anti-inflammatory activity.

Echinacea has been used in a wide variety of preparations, including ointments, lotions, creams, fluid extracts, tinctures, dry extracts, and toothpastes. Primary external uses (salves and ointments) include use as a treatment for hard-to-heal infections, wounds, sores, inflammatory skin diseases such as eczema, for minor burns, sunburn, and as a topical application to herpes sores (herpes simplex). Oral preparations, such as tinctures and extracts, are used to enhance resistance to infection, stimulate the lymphatic vascular system, and stimulate fibroblasts (cells involved in the development of connective tissue). Primary uses include enhancing or "stimulating" the body's own resistance against infections, especially in the prevention of colds and flu. If taken at the onset of symptoms, in small frequent doses every two to three hours for the first two days, it often helps to mobilize the body's own resistance to the condition (Weiss 1985).

Echinacea preparations demonstrate additional therapeutic value in a wide range of medical specialties including urology, gynecology, internal medicine, and dermatology. Recent clinical use in Europe has included the use of Echinacea products in the treatment of candidiasis, prostatitis, impetigo, upper-respiratory tract infections, tonsillitis, and other ailments or diseases.

At this time over 280 products (about half of which are homeopathic preparations,) containing *E. purpurea* and to a lesser extent, *E. angustifolia*, are available in West Germany alone. Additional products are sold in other European countries and in American markets.

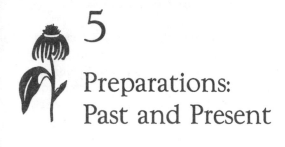

5
Preparations:
Past and Present

Over the past 100 years, Echinacea has been marketed and manufactured in a number of forms. Cut and sifted, whole and powdered roots, tinctures, and extracts (some of which are tinctures simply labeled as "extracts") of *E. angustifolia, E. pallida,* and *E. purpurea* are sold today on the American herb market. An infusion of the fresh or dried roots, powdered roots, and encapsulated dried tops of *E. purpurea* are popular preparations. Unfortunately, some manufacturers continue to include the adulterant *Parthenium integrifolium* in their products. I personally avoid "Echinacea" products which include *Parthenium integrifolium* on the list of ingredients.

Lloyd Brothers Pharmacists, Inc., were the first to manufacture a commercial Echinacea preparation of pharmaceutical quality. Their product line included Specific Medicine Echinacea, a tincture containing 69 percent alcohol; Echafolta, the trade name for a concentrated root extract excluding sugar compounds, coloring matter, chlorophyll, and other extraneous matter; Echafolta Cream, Iodized Echafolta, Aseptafolta, containing myrrh, asepin, glycerin, and Echinacea; and Subculoyd Inula and Echinacea, an injectable preparation. After experimenting with Echinacea for fourteen years, John Uri Lloyd felt a tincture of the dried root of *E. angustifolia* containing 69 percent alcohol was the best preparation.

Echinacin®, manufactured by the Madaus company of Cologne since 1939, is the oldest product form of *E. purpurea.* This extraction of the expressed fresh juice of whole flowering plants of *E. purpurea* (harvested about 8 inches above ground level) is sold in injectable, liquid extracts and in ointment form, and is also used as an ingredient in toothpastes and other products. A vast majority of the German studies on *E. purpurea* have involved Echinacin®.

Doses of Echinacea range from five to sixty drops of tincture in a little water four to six times per day. Smaller, more frequent doses (five to twenty drops) are considered best by some herbalists. Large doses can result in diminished biological activity of preparations used over the long term.

There has been some controversy over the question of whether alcohol tinctures are immunologically active, since polysaccharides precipitate out in alcohol. Other constituents besides polysaccharides are now known to be involved in immunological activity. Therefore, the point is probably moot.

Echinacea preparations once enjoyed minor acceptance in the allopathic materia medica in the United States. *E. angustifolia* or *E. pallida* were listed as official medicines in the *National Formulary* from 1916 through 1950. Uses included inducing saliva and as an alterative and diaphoretic (Vogel 1970). The mother tinctures of both *E. an-*

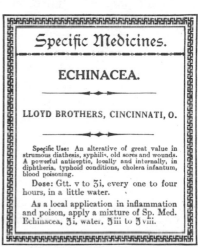

Specific Medicine Echinacea, the first pharmaceutical grade Echinacea product

gustifolia and *E. purpurea,* at 1X strength in 55 percent alcohol, are also official medicines in the 1989 supplement to the *Homeopathic Pharmacopoeia of the United States* (Homeopathic Pharmacopoeia Convention of the United States 1981, 1989).

Currently, the above-ground parts of *E. purpurea* and *E. angustifolia* are subjects of the official German monograph system for phytopharmaceuticals produced by "Commission E" of the

BGA (the German FDA). In Germany these sophisticated standard registrations for plant drugs include the name of the drug, its composition, areas of allowed application, contraindications, side effects, interactions with other drugs, dosage, mode of administration, duration of administration, and effects of the drug. In the monograph for the aerial parts of the plant, the drug is composed of preparations of the expressed juice of plant materials. No contraindications are listed for external use, though oral or injectable forms—as with all non-specific immune system stimulants—are to be used with care in autoimmune diseases, known or increased tendency to allergies, and chronic progressive infections (see chapter 6, "Safety: Risk vs. Benefits"). Echinacea is allowed to be sold as a nonspecific stimulant to the immune system to increase the body's own defenses. It does so by raising properdin levels, increasing phagocytosis, and by releasing corticosteroids. For these purposes oral and injectable forms are used. Average daily doses of oral forms are listed as 6 to 9 ml., depending upon the preparation. Dosage of injectable forms is to be determined by the physician. Externally, products are allowed to help stimulate regenerative processes, restore damaged tissue, activate phagocytosis, and for an indirect anti-infective influence resulting from the effect of the herb on the hyaluronidase/hyaluronic acid system.

Commission E in Germany has prepared nearly 300 monographs on medicinal plants. Three general categories are included. Positive monographs elucidate accepted uses. Zero or neutral monographs have been produced for drugs considered harmless but ineffectual. Negative monographs have been produced for unaccepted uses. Based on conversations with BGA officials as this book goes to press, it is possible that a negative monograph could be issued on Echinacea roots, given the confusion of identity of source material in the marketplace (see chapter 8, "Is it Echinacea?").

Is Any One Species the Best?

This question has often been heard in the herb business and among herbalists. There is an unequivocal answer: *E. purpurea* is the best species to use for the simple reason that at the present time it is the only Echinacea species for which the vast majority of the market supply is provided by cultivated rather than wild-harvested material. A naive prejudice exists, even among professional herbalists, that wild-harvested plant materials are more "active" than cultivated plants. While this may be true for ginseng, it is rarely true for other herbs. The use of *E. pallida* and *E. angustifolia* should, in my opinion, be curtailed and discouraged until the majority of the dried root of those species made available in botanical markets is supplied by cultivated rather than wild-dug material.

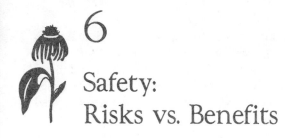

6

Safety:
Risks vs. Benefits

Echinacea is generally considered safe and nontoxic in normal dosage ranges. In his review of case histories on the use of Echinacin® in the treatment of chronic polyarthritis, D. Reuß (1986), a medical doctor who has used Echinacea preparations extensively in his general practice for over three decades, notes that he has not observed a single case of Echinacea-induced side effects in polyarthritis or other conditions for which he has employed Echinacea. However, as can be expected for ingestion or application of any substance or plant material, there are risks and benefits. While isolated adverse reactions have been reported in the use (or misuse) of Echinacea products, the long history of safe use, coupled with recent laboratory data, shows that the benefits far outweigh any inherent risks.

According to an article published in *Medical Herbalism* (1990), a new monograph on Echinacea published by the German Commission E (9 April 1990) noted contraindications for the internal use of Echinacea for known or suspected autoimmune diseases. Theoretically, as with all nonspecific immunostimulatory agents, Echinacea is contraindicated in conditions in which the immune system itself causes disease disturbances of various body tissues. For example, it is recommended that nonspecific immunostimulatory agents be used with caution for leukosis (conditions involving an abnormal proliferation of white blood cells) and in conditions known as collagenosis, in which connective tissues are attacked by the immune system (as in lupus erythematosis). Immunostimulants are generally contraindicated in multiple sclerosis (which involves a heightened immune response) and in tuberculosis (even though Echinacea has been shown to be a useful adjunct therapy for this disease). Injections or oral dosage forms are to be used cautiously in diabetes mellitus because of fears that immunostimulants may adversely affect a patient's metabolism.

Injectable forms of Echinacea preparations are contraindicated when a patient is inclined to allergies to other Compositae (aster family) members, and in pregnancy. A single isolated case of an anaphylactic reaction to injectable Echinacea drugs has been recorded, according to the Commission E monograph.

Intravenous or intramuscular dosage forms may cause self-limiting fevers or systemic reactions for a short period of time. These effects are well documented in clinical literature. No side effects are recorded for oral or locally applied dosage forms. Dosage indications suggest limiting the duration of treatment to three weeks with injectable forms, and eight weeks for oral preparations.

A 1989 paper by W. Lenk of the University of Munich reported on the acute toxicity of various fractions of polysaccharides derived both from above-ground plant parts and cell cultures of *E. purpurea*. The fractions were found to be only slightly toxic or virtually nontoxic following injections in male and female mice. The lethal dose that killed 50 percent of the animals (LD_{50}) was equal to or greater than 5000 mg/kg. In other words, it took about one-fifth of an ounce for each 2.2 pounds of body weight of the polysaccharide to produce a lethal dose, a very high amount not comparable to any therapeutic dose of the substance. In short, the polysaccharides were found to be virtually nontoxic.

Such animal studies raise a number of ethical questions. The safety of Echinacea is well documented in the clinical experience of dozens of physicians over the past 100 years. However, as Reuß (1986) notes, unfortunately the doctor's accurate observations of the patient do not count for much in assessing the results of a treatment. It is randomized, double-blind studies or laboratory parameters with extensive statistical analysis that are significant—not empirical observations.

A 1978 German law grandfathered the sale of phytopharmaceuticals for a twelve-year period, after which such products have to be proven safe and effective using the standards of Western medicine. As a result, in the 1980s we began to see more laboratory-based pharmacological and toxicological studies along with double-blind clinical trials to justify the use of medicinal plant products (including Echinacea) under standards set forth for the acceptance of synthetic Western drugs.

At the same time, however, traditional animal studies are under attack. A number of researchers, both in West Germany and the United States have expressed to me that given the growing negative attitude toward animal studies, it is actually less difficult to obtain permission to conduct human trails on a substance which has a reasonable certainty of safety than it is to receive permission to develop animal studies. Western researchers often focus on proving *if* a medicinal plant is safe and effective. In China, on the other hand, with a long continuous history of medicinal plant use, safety and efficacy are well documented and accepted. In China, Western-style pharmacological and safety studies focus on *how* the medicinal plant works. Given the growing problems and ethical questions surrounding animal research in the West, many biological researchers are developing more studies based on laboratory cell cultures.

A paper by O. Schimmer, G. Abel, and C. Behninger of the University of Erlangen-Nürnberg, published in 1989, reported on the genotoxic potency of a polysaccharide (a neutral fucogalactoxyloglucan) from *E. purpurea* cell culture using cultured human lymphocytes. Even in low concentrations, the substance did not affect the lymphocytes in any adverse manner, including their ability to reproduce, providing further evidence of the safety of the active polysaccharides of *E. purpurea*.

These recent studies further confirm the long-held recognition of the safety of Echinacea. Safe use generally means rational use. Problems have resulted from inappropriate self-administration of Echinacea products for acute conditions. For example, a strong tincture of *E. angustifolia* should not be applied directly to irritated, inflamed mucous membrane surfaces, such as a severe sore throat. One case came to the author's attention in which a tincture was dropped directly into a severely infected ear, resulting in aggravation of the condition. While oral dosage, coupled with antibiotics, may have helped the condition, direct application of the tincture was more harmful than helpful. Digestive irritations can be mitigated by administering Echinacea tinctures in a little water rather than taking it full strength.

In most cases of self-medication, Echinacea products work best at the onset of symptoms for acute minor skin irritations, sores, colds, and flu, rather than when symptoms are fully developed. They are used for a three- to five day period; then use is discontinued until needed again. There is evidence that the positive preventive effect for acute viral infections diminishes after three days. Echinacea should be taken as needed, rather than on a continuous basis. In Europe, pharmaceutical drug preparations containing Echinacea may be administered by a health care practitioner for more serious conditions (nonself-limiting conditions).

Other sensitivities have been reported in dermatological patch tests, homeopathic provings, and in excessive use of *E. angustifolia*. According to James A. Duke, "In Mitchell and Rooks' *Dermatology* (1979) we read that Echinacea, which was a constituent of a proprietary remedy, produced positive patch test reactions in four patients who had previously suffered plant dermatitis. . . ." (Duke 1979).

Homeopathic provings have been conducted in order to establish symptoms for which Echinacea may be effective in ultramolecular homeopathic doses. Hepburn *et al.* (1950) administered *E. angustifolia* tincture in 8 minim doses over thirteen days, which produced excessive thirst, perspiration, and fluctuations in blood sugar, chlorides, and blood cholesterol levels.

Bruce Canvasser (in Sherman 1979) reports *E. angustifolia* may cause headaches, joint pains, gastrointestinal disturbances, and dry tongue.

If Echinacea is to become more widely available to a broader public, we must establish safe and effective uses of Echinacea products. We must also establish a sustainable source of supply, identify means of assuring that the plant material in a product container is the same as what the label claims, and lastly, provide a means of assuring that the genetic information in wild populations will be maintained and conserved for the survival of the biodiversity of the genus Echinacea. I believe that these three adjunct but integral problems to the future development of the medicinal use of Echinacea can largely be overcome by establishing cultivated supplies of Echinacea species used in the manufacture of products.

7

On the Farm and in the Garden: Cultivating Echinacea

Echinacea purpurea has been cultivated as a hardy, showy, perennial garden ornamental since the early 1700s, both in North America and Europe. It is easily grown from seed, is drought tolerant, will grow in full sun or partial shade, and thrives on neglect. *Echinacea pallida* is commonly planted in prairie restoration projects, meadow lawn plantings, and sometimes in herb gardens. The yellow-flowered *E. paradoxa* was introduced to the horticultural trade by this writer in 1984. At least three nurseries now sell seed or plants of this handsome perennial. Three Tennessee nurseries are licensed to sell the unusual, attractive, endangered perennial, *E. tennesseensis*. The Narrow-Leaved Purple Coneflower *E. angustifolia* is primarily grown by collectors of medicinal plants. A handful of small commercial plantings are in place. *Echinacea simulata* has been offered in the horticultural trade (often as *E. pallida*). *Echinacea atrorubens, E. laevigata,* and *E. sanguinea* are rarely seen in cultivation.

Accessing the Genetic Code: Propagation

Echinaceas are not that difficult to propagate, but be forewarned, it's not as easy as starting tomatoes. Echinacea can be started from seeds, by dividing offshoots of the crowns, or by planting 4- to 5-inch sections of the roots (as you would with comfrey).

There are a few tricks to growing Echinacea from seed that will help to ensure success. Echinacea seeds are embryo dormant, and a period of cold moist stratification greatly increases the speed and frequency of germination. Seeds can be placed in a mix of sand and peat and placed outdoors (covered with a mesh screen to keep critters out) and left over the winter.

Another way is to place seeds in moist but not wet sand (or peat) in a plastic bag and refrigerate for one to four months (duration depending upon species). Once the stratification period is completed, simply wash the seeds in a strainer to remove the sand. The mesh of the strainer must be smaller than the seeds, yet large enough for the sand to pass through.

Planting seeds on top of the soil mix, then tamping them down on the soil surface, will generally result in quicker germination than if the seeds are planted beneath the soil surface. In the uncontrolled environment of a home windowsill, seeds of *E. purpurea,* stratified for one month then sown on the surface of a soil mix (⅓ sand, ⅓ peat, ⅓ sterile potting soil), germinated within five days after planting. Those seeds that were covered with about ⅛ inch of soil germinated in two weeks to a month. The seeds were placed in a south-facing window and subjected to the variable temperature and humidity conditions of a house heated exclusively with a wood stove. The germination rate was about 50 percent. Parallel results were observed in germinating seeds of *E. pallida, E. simulata, E. paradoxa,* and *E. angustifolia,* stratified under varying time periods.

Echinacea seed can also be sown directly in the garden in the fall, though germination rates are usually substantially lower than greenhouse or cold frame-sown seeds. If seeds are planted outdoors, they should be protected with a straw mulch.

Salac, Traeger, and Jensen (1982) have shown that the establishment of plants is enhanced by planting seedlings in the field or by transplanting cuttings. They further showed that seed tamped into the soil surface germinated in five days. Seed covered with ⅛ inch of soil took two to four weeks to germinate. Germination rates were much higher with cold frame or greenhouse grown seedlings compared with those directly sown in the field.

A study done by Thomas E. Hemmerly (1976) as a doctoral dissertation at Vanderbilt University shows that the longer stratification period results in an increase in both frequency and percentage of germination. His tests included seeds of *E. tennesseensis*, *E. pallida*, and *E. purpurea*. The *E. purpurea* seeds showed their highest germination rates after ten rather than sixteen weeks of stratification.

Hemmerly's studies showed that stratification and temperature were the most important factors in the germination of the three Echinacea species he studied. The longer the stratification period (up to four months), the less important temperature became as a factor in seed germination. Light was found to be a germination-stimulating or promoting factor, though much less significant than temperature and stratification. The optimum temperature for germinating Echinacea seed under light is around 20° to 25° C (about 68° to 79° F).

I have attempted to stratify *E. angustifolia* for four months in the uncontrolled conditions of the home refrigerator, but found that after ninty days the seeds began to sprout in the stratification medium. Based on my own experience, a sixty to ninty day stratification period for *E. angustifolia* seems adequate, under household rather than laboratory conditions.

However, a study published by the Agricultural Experiment Station of the University of Nebraska, Lincoln, (Ottoson, 1978) suggests the optimum germination rate (49 percent) for *E. angustifolia* occurred after a stratification period of fifteen weeks at 39.2° F (4° C), coupled with a photoperiod of 14.5 hours light, and 9.5 hours dark. The germination temperature was 78° F (26° C).

Various reports on the germination of Echinacea seed have appeared in journals dealing with prairie ecology. Blake (1935) found that germination of *E. angustifolia* seed increased by 36 percent if seed was stratified naturally before planting. Hesse (1973) showed that artificial stratification for fifteen weeks at 4° C increased germination of seeds at 19° C or 26° C. When the corky seed covering of *E. angustifolia* was removed, Sorensen and Holden (1974) reported a 79 percent increase in germination of nonstratified seed.

Smith-Jochum (1987) studied germination requirements, field

cultivation, and field establishment of *E. angustifolia, E. purpurea,* and *E. pallida.* In all species, her study showed that one month stratification in peat moss or sand, twenty-four hour water soak and control (no treatment) showed significantly higher germination rates than two months stratification in sand or peat moss with soaking for twenty-four hours in potassium nitrate or treatment with gibberelic acid.

In field planting, fall sowing in flat beds gave the highest field germination rates for *E. purpurea* and *E. pallida. Echinacea pallida* showed better fall emergence than *E. purpurea. Echinacea purpurea,* however, showed better spring emergence than *E. pallida.* The greenhouse germination rate of *E. purpurea* was significantly higher than the other two species tested. Greenhouse establishment of seedlings, which were then transplanted into permanent beds, proved to enhance seedling development over directly seeded fall plantings.

Smith-Jochum's studies also focused on quantity and quality of essential oil content. She concluded that *E. pallida* produced higher levels of essential oil than *E. angustifolia* and *E. purpurea.* Fall transplanting and harvest seemed to produce both greater quantity and quality (based on gas-liquid chromatography peaks) of essential oil.

Hipps (1988) suggests that slicing off the petal end of *E. purpurea* seed may enhance germination without stratification. Rick Grazzini (1988a) of H. G. German Seeds, Smethport, Pennsylvania, learned this technique from a USDA botanist who specialized in *Rudbeckia* back in the 1950s. It simply involves "clipping" or slicing off the pappus (reduced to a smooth or toothed crown in the genus Echinacea) at the "petal end" (distal or "fat" end) of Echinacea seed. However, only a little sliver at the very crown would work, otherwise one cuts into, and damages, the cotyledon. This technique shows promise for future studies on Echinacea seed germination. R. Grazzini (1988b) theorizes that perhaps the seeds harbor a water-soluble germination inhibitor, and that clipping the petal end simply allows the theoretical germination inhibitor to leach out at a faster rate.

Grazzini's firm is working with other horticultural companies to study a technique known as "priming" to enhance germination potential of *E. purpurea*. The seeds are soaked to imbibe water until a certain osmotic moisture potential is achieved, then the moisture level is reduced to a predetermined optimum level. This technique may not only enhance availability of *E. purpurea* in the greenhouse trade, but if successful, might be the key to unlocking germination enhancement of *E. angustifolia,* making it viable to germinate seeds for commercial plantings. As a conservation tool to develop larger-scale propagation and cultivation, this technique might conceivably be applied to the endangered *E. tennesseensis* and *E. laevigata.*

While it has previously been stated that Echinacea seeds are embryo dormant and need to be stratified for optimum germination, the mechanism of seed dormancy in Echinacea is poorly understood. Do Echinacea species have a physiologically inactive embryo or germination inhibitors such as aldehydes, ethylenes, acids, phyto-hormones, or other compounds? Do the seeds have an immature or rudimentary embryo? Do they have combined dormancy including several germination-inhibiting factors?

Another factor in determining experimental germination per-centages in Echinacea is whether low germination is due to dor-mancy, unfilled (empty) seeds, or dead seeds (with aborted embryos). It has been recommended that all ungerminated seeds of aster fam-ily members be examined at the end of testing to determine whether those seeds are dead, empty, or dormant (USDA, 1952). More gen-eral studies on physiology, biology, and chemistry of Echinacea seeds are sorely needed.

One pound of *E. angustifolia* seeds contains about 145,000 seeds. Seeds remain viable in dry cold storage for at least sixty months (Ottoson, 1978). There are approximately 117,000 seeds in a pound of *E. purpurea,* and seed can be sown at a rate of twelve pounds per acre (broadcast). If seedlings are started in a greenhouse, then planted at 1.5-foot intervals with rows spaced three feet apart, an acre should hold about 9,800 plants. Even with a poor germination rate, one pound of seed should be sufficient to plant an acre with ease.

Seed for *E. purpurea* and seedlings of its cultivars are readily available on the horticultural trade. Bulk prices for *E. purpurea* seed range from $30 to $90 per pound. Seeds and seedlings of *E. pallida* can be obtained from sources specializing in prairie restoration. Seed and plant sources of *E. angustifolia* are more difficult to find. *Echinacea pallida* seed and plants have sometimes been offered as *E. angustifolia* (see appendix).

Once seedlings are six to seven weeks old, they can be transplanted to a permanent location. Vegetative development is very slow the first year. Don't expect the plants to get much larger than they were after eight weeks of growth, especially for slow-growing *E. angustifolia,* which often flowers in the second or third year. *Echinacea purpurea,* on the other hand, may grow rapidly and flower the first year, though it usually takes two years to flower. Weed control is very important, since the young seedlings do not do well in a highly competitive environment.

Echinacea can also be propagated by dividing offshoots from the crowns. Once you've gone to the effort of growing the plant for two to four years, there is no sense killing the plant once the root is harvested. After harvesting the root, the top half-inch or inch (including the crown) can be replanted. Depending upon the age of the root, you should be able to divide two to seven buds or "eyes" from one crown. Each bud can produce a new plant. If roots are harvested in the late fall, the roots can be heeled in sand in a root cellar for the winter months, as one might do for root crops such as carrots or parsnips. Make sure you keep the sand moist through the winter. The root crowns may then be planted in the spring. If you harvest the roots in the spring while the plant is still dormant, the root crowns can be planted directly in the garden or in a cold frame as soon as dug. However, the survival rate for spring-dug crown re-growth seems to be less than that of fall-dug roots. Water the crowns occasionally until new vegetative growth is well-established. Do not expect success with this technique if you harvest the roots while vegetative growth is in progress.

Soil and Habitat

In their native habitats, *E. angustifolia* and *E. pallida* are often found growing on disturbed roadside limestone outcrops, often with high clay content. *E. purpurea* is found growing in moderately rich soil along creek beds, or in seepage, often under dappled shade. The Echinaceas are essentially lime-loving plants, though they will tolerate a slightly acid soil with a pH of 6.0 or greater. *E. angustifolia* seems to like a more alkaline soil than the other Echinacea species, a pH of around 8 being suitable. Spot checks of wild *E. simulata* habitats in the Ozarks of north central Arkansas have shown pH ranges between 4.5 to 8.0, though over 80 percent of the samples taken had pH ranges between 5.9 to 7.0.

Echinaceas are exceptionally drought tolerant. William J. Dress states that his *E. purpurea* stands up to droughty conditions better than any other perennial in his garden (personal communication 1983). A poor to moderately rich, well-drained soil will suit Echinaceas. Good soil drainage and frequent, shallow cultivation produce more vigorous plants.

Harvest and Yields

Plants grown from seeds, if roots are desired, may take three to four years to reach maturity. However, Lon Johnson of Trout Lake Farm, a commercial grower of certified organic Echinacea, suggests that older roots may become pithy and woody, and thus less desirable. Those species with tap roots will develop larger and deeper roots the longer they are in the ground. One-sixth acre of three-year-old *E. purpurea* yielded Lon Johnson 200 pounds of dried root (1,200 pounds per acre).

Fall is the best time to harvest roots, as the moisture content will usually be lower in autumn than in spring. Roots should be cleaned after they are dug, then dried under low, forced heat or dried in open air under shade.

In recent years, the tops of flowering *E. purpurea* have come under increasing demand as a commodity. If the tops of Echinacea are desired, a strong perennial planting will take two years to become established, and could produce for up to ten years. However, it is best to replace the planting every three years, rotating the crop with nitrogen-fixing legumes.

More Questions than Answers

There is still much to learn about the germplasm, chemotaxonomy, cultivation, harvesting, and storage of Echinacea which can ultimately identify the highest quality source of Echinacea root and methods for producing and preparing it. In recent years, research has shown that many factors of concern to the grower determine the quality of plant medicines. Within a given species there may be chemical variation, in certain populations due to subtle genetic differences that are undetectable upon visual inspection; environmental differences affecting quality (such as soil and climate condition), or chemical differences in various plant parts at different stages of growth.

Studies with both Foxglove and the Opium Poppy demonstrate that their active chemical constituents are most highly concentrated at certain stages in the plants' development. In the Opium Poppy, morphine content peaks two to three weeks after flowering. If similar studies were conducted on Echinacea, interesting findings might result.

How do different soil types affect the quality of Echinacea? Plants growing in dry, low-nitrogen soils produce higher concentrations of essential oils, while moist, nitrogen-rich soils produce higher levels of alkaloids.

The time of day a plant is harvested can also affect the quality of chemical constituents and their concentrations in various plant parts, as can weather conditions.

Manufacturers of pharmaceutical-grade botanical preparations avoid rapid drying of essential oil-containing plants (and slow drying of plants with cardiac glycosides, like Foxglove), because these drying methods may significantly lower the amount of active constituents. Slow drying of Foxglove is avoided because the glycosides are rapidly hydrolyzed by enzymes. *Echinacea angustifolia* contains a glucoside and an essential oil, both of which contribute to its pharmacological activity.

Genetic and environmental differences in populations of *E. angustifolia* may explain why John Uri Lloyd preferred roots from a certain region of Nebraska. Individual plants from the same population in a given locality could develop into chemical races which may produce a higher quality Echinacea product. It is very important, therefore, to preserve the genetic diversity of Echinacea species by protecting wild populations. It is possible that one wild harvester could wipe out an important chemical race in one day. Preservation must become a prime consideration of wild harvesters and commercial buyers of Echinacea and other medicinal plants. Unfortunately, these words ring hollow, because since the first edition of this publication appeared in 1983, we have seen even greater stress on wild Echinacea populations.

To a great extent, the development of Echinacea as an agricultural commodity will depend upon the nuances of supply and demand. If market prices for *E. purpurea* are around $3 to $5 per pound wholesale and a farmer is able to realize a price of $3 per pound and gets a good crop of 1,200 pounds per acre after having it in the ground for three years, that farmer will gross only $1,200 per acre for each year the crop is in the ground. This is not a great incentive for most farmers to give up a known crop for an obscure crop with a specialized and uncertain market. Besides, at current consumption levels, the entire domestic market, as well as current export levels, could probably be supplied with less than 200 acres of cultivated material.

The integrity of Echinacea as a valuable medicinal plant, as well as a farm commodity, is also dependent upon knowing that when you buy Echinacea it is Echinacea that you get. The following chapter raises questions regarding the identity of some plant material that has been sold as Echinacea.

8

Is It Echinacea? Substitution and Adulteration

A rose may be a rose, but not all "Echinacea" is Echinacea. In 1985 researchers at the University of Munich (R. Bauer, I. A. Kahn, H. Lotter, and H. Wagner 1985a, 1985b), published on the discovery and elucidation of four new cinnamoyl esters of sesquiterpene alcohols in *E. purpurea*. They named them echinadiol, epoxyechinadiol, echinaxanthol, and dihydroxynardol. An article on HPLC (high pressure liquid chromatography) and TLC (thin layer chromatography) standards for the identification of *E. purpurea* and *E. angustifolia,* noting the presence of these chemical components was authored by R. Bauer, I. Kahn and H. Wagner (1986).

However, in late summer 1986, Dr. Bauer discovered that the plant material used for the studies was in fact a widespread adulterant to commercial *E. purpurea* lots, a plant known botanically as *Parthenium integrifolium.*

Parthenium integrifolium, traded as Missouri Snake Root and known by the common names Cutting Almond, Nephretic Plant, Wild Quinine, American Feverfew, and Prairie Dock, is a member of the aster family. It occurs along roadsides, on granite and limestone outcrops, and in prairies and open woods from Massachusetts to Georgia, west to Texas, and north to Minnesota. Five distinct varieties are recognized (Mears 1975). Historically, it has been used as a diuretic for bladder and kidney ailments, gonorrhea, and as a stimulant and an aromatic bitter. The flowering tops were once used for intermittent fevers (such as malaria), hence the common names American Feverfew and Wild Quinine (Foster 1987a). The live plant at any stage of growth looks nothing like any species of Echinacea.

Though Parthenium is not similar in appearance to Echinacea, once the root is cut and sifted it has an uncanny resemblance to *E. angustifolia* or *E. pallida* roots, though it possesses its own characteristic flavor and fragrance. It does not resemble the root of *E. purpurea*. One Parthenium root may weigh ten times more than one *E. purpurea* root.

Parthenium has been documented as an adulterant in commercial Echinacea lots as early as 1909 (Moser 1910). John Uri Lloyd (1924) noted that Echinacea was one of the most variable drugs known to him in its crude form, and he found that insipid, tasteless lots of Echinacea root had little medicinal value. Other adulterants in lots of the dried root mentioned by J. U. Lloyd included *Lespedeza capitata* (Round-headed Bush Clover), *Eryngium aquaticum* (Rattlesnake-master), *Rudbeckia nitida* (St. John's-susan), *Helianthus annuus* (Common Sunflower), *Liatris aspera* (Rough Blazing Star), and unidentified plant roots.

The present author noted the presence of *P. integrifolium* as a "substitute" to modern commercial lots of *E. purpurea* in a short 1985 article, "Herb Traders Beware," in *HerbalGram* (Foster 1985a). The problem was again mentioned in another 1985 article, "Echinacea— An Honest Appraisal" (1985b). The subject was further discussed in the second edition of *Echinacea Exalted* (1985d).

The latter publication was sent to R. Bauer and H. Wagner in June of 1986. In July of that year R. Bauer requested voucher specimens of *P. integrifolium* for chemical comparison, which were sent in August of 1986. Subsequently R. Bauer and his colleagues at the University of Munich confirmed the appearance of *P. integrifolium* in commercial lots of *E. purpurea* in Europe by comparing authenticated specimens provided by this author, the Herbarium of the Botanical Institute, Munich, and Munich Botanical Garden. This investigation by R. Bauer, I. Khan, K. Jurcic, and H. Wagner (1986) was presented as a poster at the Phytochemical Society of Europe's 1986 meeting in Lausanne, Switzerland.

Bauer's purpose (personal communication, 23–26 April 1987) in performing the 1985 chemical study on *E. purpurea* was to look at the chemistry of commercial *E. purpurea* products. An assumption was made that the plant material in the marketplace was correctly labeled. That assumption proved erroneous. About twenty different batches of commercial *"E. purpurea"* roots were tested which showed four characteristic patterns in chemical assay. Isolation and elucidation of the chemical structure yielded four new compounds. Further study showed that the work had in fact been done on *P. integrifolium* root products labeled *E. purpurea*.

It was only after testing fresh roots of vouchered specimens of *E. purpurea* that Dr. Rudolf Bauer's research group was able to ascertain the extent of the problem. Chemical fingerprints of vouchered specimens of *P. integrifolium* produced the same results as the commercial samples on which these researchers had originally published their results. It was further shown that the adulteration problem only existed with roots imported from the United States. There was no question as to the identity of commercial supplies of *E. purpurea* grown in Europe. These researchers also found samples of *E. angustifolia* adulterated with *P. integrifolium*. The present author has also seen several products labeled as *"E. angustifolia"* which contained Parthenium root.

Bauer and his associates at the University of Munich published several articles on how to identify true *E. purpurea* and *P. integrifolium* using chemical fingerprints, so that other researchers and herb companies could determine the presence of the adulterant. An ironic twist to the story was that Bauer's preliminary pharmacological studies indicated that one or more of the chemical components he isolated from Parthenium very well *may* possess some immuno-stimulating activity. The studies were preliminary and should not be inflated out of context.

Furthermore, according to Bauer, the genus Parthenium is well-known for its allergenic properties, and believes that the examination of *E. purpurea* root for adulteration with *P. integrifolium* should be compulsory.

This was not the first case of mistaken identity of Echinacea imported to Germany from the United States. After the 1930s, very little Echinacea was sold on the American market and there was virtually no demand for *E. purpurea*; therefore, adulteration was not a problem. Most Echinacea products sold at that time which were labeled *E. angustifolia* contained correctly identified plant material or *E. pallida*. *Echinacea purpurea* itself does not appear to have been traded in commercial botanical markets until the 1930s, when the Madaus company of Cologne began to develop its Echinacin® product.

According to Dr. Bauer (personal communication, 23–26 April 1987), the Madaus company had originally intended to cultivate *E. angustifolia* in Germany and had ordered several pounds of the seed from a United States seed company. They received seed labeled *"E. angustifolia,"* but the plants which grew from the seeds turned out to be *E. purpurea*. Desiring to grow their own supply of cultivated Echinacea, the company performed research and developed its product from *E. purpurea*. While *E. purpurea* is the earliest Echinacea species mentioned in medicinal plant literature, it has been commercially developed (supported by a large body of scientific literature) only in the past sixty years. The identity of the plant material used in the manufacture of the Madaus Echinacin® product has never been in question.

According to Bauer, Khan, and Wagner (1987), the presence of Parthenium as an adulterant in the German market was mentioned as early as 1952 by Stoll and Seebeck. Hobbs (1989) notes that in 1957, F. Auster and J. Schafer also warned of the potential adulterant problem in Germany.

The identity of the plant material used in many studies on the pharmacology and clinical applications of *E. purpurea* is not in question. According to Hobbs (1989) a large majority of the clinical studies have involved two products manufactured in Germany from freshly harvested *E. purpurea* grown in that country. In addition, a number of manufacturers of tinctures and extracts and small commercial growers of dried *E. purpurea* root in the United States have had properly identified and labeled plant material from the outset. Their products, too, are not in question.

In fact, any cultivated *E. purpurea* source is not involved in the Parthenium substitution equation. *Echinacea purpurea* never occurs in the wild in quantities suitable for commercial harvest. There is no wild-harvested *E. purpurea* on world markets. Cultivated material can be easily identified and verified from the original source.

By the time Echinacea products began to gain popularity in the United States during the 1980s, the substitution problem came to the attention of the herb industry. It soon became clear that much of what was being sold at the time under the trade name of "Missouri Snake Root" and labeled *"Echinacea purpurea"* was in fact *P. integrifolium.*

According to Mark Blumenthal, publisher of *HerbalGram*, and executive director of the American Botanical Council, Austin, Texas, "It was a problem—and still is—until all companies acknowledge the problem exists and move to correct it. We have seen several companies in good faith move fairly quickly to get adequate supplies of authenticated material, but the possibility exists that some companies have not yet fully acknowledged the importance of doing so. This further underscores the need for using scientific or botanical names in the labeling of herb products. If all companies had used botanical names on their products, the problem would not have become so widespread" (personal communication 1987).

The substitution problem produced a difficult situation for commercial growers of *E. purpurea,* both in Europe and the United States, as well as manufacturers of Echinacea products which contained authentic *E. purpurea.* One grower affected was Lon Johnson of Trout Lake Farm. Trout Lake has over thirty acres of three species of Echinacea under cultivation for the production of bulk dried Echinacea leaves, roots, and seeds. Florammune, a fresh plant tincture (alcohol extract) of *E. purpurea* and *E. angustifolia,* is manufactured nearby from plants grown at Trout Lake Farm. Based on the growing popularity of the herb, Johnson had planted several acres of *E. purpurea,* but had a difficult time selling the dried root at a price high enough to cover production costs, in part due to the presence of the high-weight, low-priced Parthenium roots in commercial markets.

"We had a good year in 1987 anticipating demand and increased our production, but we would have fallen flat on our faces if we had done it before. If we increased our acreage much more now, we would again face problems for that increase in supply as well. There was cultivated *E. purpurea* out there that we could have harvested, if more demand had surfaced, and there is a potential for that in the future.

"The bottom line in whether an herbal medicine is effective," Johnson says, "is directly related to the quality of the herbs. We cannot expect results with herbal medicine, obviously, unless the quality is high. Consumers have a right to assume an inherent quality in herbal products. They assume that the plant material is properly identified and that the ingredients make sense. They do not expect ingredients that are the result of some kind of historical mistake, apology, or market dependence. Some companies aren't looking for a supply of properly identified Echinacea, even though they know where to get it. *Parthenium integrifolium* is just not found in the historical herbal or scientific literature and people shouldn't be swayed into buying something as an Echinacea product that has Echinacea way down on the list of ingredients, with Parthenium as the main ingredient. If Echinacea is a minor ingredient, it doesn't make the product an Echinacea product" (personal communication 1987).

The situation prompted the Standards Committee of the American Herbal Products Association (AHPA) to look into instituting a program of product testing. AHPA is a trade association serving herb product manufacturers. The AHPA program not only applies to Echinacea products, but to any other herb commodities that may suffer from identity or mislabeling problems. AHPA will attempt to identify all companies selling the products or ingredients in question, who will then be offered the opportunity to participate in a testing program. The program to test Echinacea products will involve sending product samples to independent laboratories for identification and verification of the Echinacea contents.

According to AHPA Standards Committee Chairman Timothy Moley, before the labs are selected, they will be sent blind samples of the plant materials to test the lab's ability to properly identify the plant. The lab's ability will also be periodically tested by the submission of reference samples.

Unfortunately, because of various factors and complications, the AHPA program is not yet in place. However, in bringing the issue to the attention of its members, AHPA did much to alter the market situation in a positive way.

Some companies, however, have persisted in using *P. integrifolium* root as a base for "Echinacea" products.

Those searching for detailed scientific information on the identification of *E. angustifolia, E. pallida, E. purpurea,* and *P. integrifolium* using chemical analytical methods are referred to the following articles (in German unless otherwise noted): Bauer, Khan and Wagner 1987; Bauer, Remiger and Wagner 1988; Bauer, Khan and Wagner 1988 (in English); Bauer and Remiger 1989a; and Bauer and Remiger 1989b (in English). Information on microscopic identification of the four species can be found in Heubl and Bauer 1989; and Heubl, Bauer and Wagner 1989.

HPLC (high pressure liquid chromatography) and TLC (thin layer chromatography) analysis of *E. purpurea* and *P. integrifolium* can be determined on the basis of the sesquiterpene esters of the *P. integrifolium,* and the caffeic acid derivatives of *E. purpurea* (Bauer, Khan, and Wagner 1987). Comparative HPLC and TLC fingerprint standards have also been developed for *E. purpurea, E. angustifolia,* and *E. pallida.* The hydroxycinnamic acid derivatives of the three species were significantly different, as were quantities of cichoric acid, though the content of isobutylamides was quite similar (Bauer, Remiger and Wagner 1988a).

Previously published articles on the microscopic identification of Echinacea included Gathercoal and Wirth (1949), Kraemer and

Sollenberger (1911), and Kraemer (1912). These are reviewed by Foster (1987a) and Hobbs (1989). Hobbs provides details of HPLC and TLC analysis of Echinacea species vs. Parthenium translated from the German literature.

As was previously noted, commercial lots of *E. angustifolia* have long been adulterated with *E. pallida.* This was chemically confirmed in comparing commercial samples of root products of both species with more than ten batches of authentic voucher specimens of the roots supplied by eight botanists or growers. The roots of both species contain different primary constituents, and those of *E. pallida* are unstable in storage. Furthermore, both species have been shown to contain echinacoside, which in the past was said to be a chemical marker for *E. angustifolia,* and had been used in the identification of that species. This can no longer be the case (Bauer, Khan, and Wagner 1988).

In a recent study, it has also been shown that echinacoside also occurs in *E. simulata* and *E. paradoxa.* Therefore, the presence of this constituent cannot be used to distinguish between various Echinacea species (Bauer and Foster 1989). Without the availability of reference voucher specimens for previous chemical studies on *E. angustifolia,* one cannot be sure which species was actually used; thus the results must be questioned.

What should the consumer do? Certainly he or she is not in a position to reference German scientific literature on the chemical and microscopic analysis of Echinacea products. Consumers are warned to read the list of ingredients. If *P. integrifolium* or the trade name "Missouri Snake Root" appears on the list of ingredients in an Echinacea product, I personally avoid that product. Since virtually no *E. purpurea* is harvested from the wild, those products which contain "certified organic" *E. purpurea* can generally be assumed to be a correctly identified, cultivated product, grown without the use of pesticides. Unfortunately, several manufacturers label their product "organic" without the product being certified by a third-party certification organization. The use of the term "organic" in labeling has specific legal implications in about half of the states. Federal regulations providing a national definition of "organic" in product labeling are being drafted by the Congress as this book goes to press.

Removing the adulterant from the marketplace, coupled with increased demand for Echinacea products, poses yet another problem: conserving wild populations of Echinacea. The last chapter outlines the conservation issues relative to Echinacea. Could Echinacea be developed for other commercial products besides those used in human medicine? The following chapter deals with other uses of the plant group.

9

A Natural Insecticide for the Future?

Some chemical components evolve in plants as a kind of insect repellent to thwart attacks from potential predators. Since the 1940s hundreds of plant species have been studied as potential sources of new compounds that might have insecticidal components. With growing public dislike for synthetic pesticides, more scientists are turning to plants as a potential source of insecticides that could be used with success on important crops, yet have minimal impact on the environment. Echinacea is one of the plant groups that has been studied, starting with a 1947 report by A. Hartzell, which found that acetone extracts of Echinacea killed 50 percent of the larvae of a mosquito *(Culex quinquefasciatus)* at concentrations of 1000 ppm or less.

Martin Jacobson, a USDA researcher (1954, 1967) isolated echinacein, an insecticidal component in Echinacea root, which was found to be effective against the adult housefly, the German cockroach, and the yellow mealworm. Jacobson, Redfern and Mills (1975) isolated echinolone, an insect-growth regulator mimicking juvenile hormones in the yellow meal worm. Bame (1984) showed that an extract of echinacein was toxic to the western corn rootworm larvae.

In recent years, researchers in the Horticulture Department at South Dakota State University attempted to identify Echinacea varieties containing the highest levels of echinolone to develop an insecticide to use on the state's sunflower crop. Twenty-five percent of the crop is lost to infestations of the northern corn fruit worm.

According to botanist Dr. Gerald A. Myers, they have been performing anatomical studies on Echinacea using electron microscopy in order to discover the exact placement of the insecticidal component in the cell structure of the plant (Kessler 1987).

Caster and Myers (1987) performed a study to establish a relationship between echinacein and oleoresins, plus locate storage, transport and synthesis sites of oleoresin in *E. purpurea.* Since the isobutylamide known as echinacein has a strong numbing effect on the tongue, taste tests determined that the highest concentrations were in the seeds and root. The numbing sensation increased with the age of the plant. The highest concentration of oleoresin canals was found in the placental region of the receptacle. The canals continued into the bracts and achenes and, according to the authors, became larger and more frequent as the flower head matured. Tissue samples of the root, leaf, floral bract, and receptacle were observed under an electron microscope. A probable relationship between the occurrence of echinacein and the presence of the oleoresin canals was established by the researchers.

Since isobutylamides are apparently involved in the immunostimulant activity of the plant as well as insecticidal activity, this research suggests that the best time for harvest of the whole fresh plant is at floral maturity.

Myers also believes that certain genes may control the insecticidal components, and that perhaps those genes could be isolated and transferred to sunflowers, producing an insect-resistant crop. Another possibility is developing the drought- and insect-resistant perennial Echinacea as an oil seed crop itself, as about 30 percent of the seed is a high-quality oil.

However, Meyer's work is posed only as representing theoretical possibilities, since funding for the Echinacea studies at South Dakota State University was eclipsed in favor of higher-priority research projects. Research continues into the chemistry of Echinacea, in hopes of discovering new compounds. A review of some of those findings is presented next.

10
Chemical Constituents

Chemical constituents of the genus Echinacea considered most important for medicinal activity include the volatile oil, the isobutylamides, the polyines and polyenes, the polysaccharides (in water extracts), cichoric acid, and the caffeic acid derivatives. Echinacoside, one caffeic acid derivative, as explained earlier, while once believed to be a significant component, probably plays a minor role in medicinal activity. It is found in four of five species tested for the component, not just in *E. angustifolia,* as once thought. Cynarine was thought to be unique to *E. angustifolia,* and Bauer has noted that it might be used as a chemical marker for this species. This substance, however, has recently been discovered in *E. tennesseensis* (see below).

These components vary in concentration depending upon the species, plant part, and other variables. As is the case with most plants, there are numerous ubiquitous components such as sugars, fatty acids, flavonoids, sterols, and other compound groups that are believed to be of little importance in the medicinal activity of the genus. Bauer and Wagner (1988) and Bauer, Khan, and Wagner (1988) also note that many previous chemical (as well as pharmacological) studies on *"E. angustifolia"* failed to distinguish between it and *E. pallida,* and therefore the results must be questioned.

The essential oil content of the roots of *E. pallida* is higher than that of the roots of *E. angustifolia* and *E. purpurea.* Bauer, Khan, and Wagner (1988) attribute this to the large amounts of polyine and polyene compounds occurring in *E. pallida.* These compounds undergo oxidation in storage, changing their composition.

Isobutylamides, the substances responsible for the numbing,

anesthetic, or "buzz factor" effect of Echinacea, are primarily components of the roots of *E. purpurea,* and *E. angustifolia,* though they are in very low concentrations in *E. pallida.* According to Jacobson (1967) echinacein, an isobutylamide comprises 0.01 percent of the dried root of *E. angustifolia* and 0.001 percent of the dried root of *E. pallida.* Jacobson (1954) notes that echinacein may be identical to neoherculin from the bark of *Zanthoxylum clava-herculis.* Jacobson, Redfern, and Mills (1975) also identified echinolone, a polyacetylene compound from *E. angustifolia,* which has potential insecticidal activity as reported in the previous chapter.

Components from fresh plant parts of *E. purpurea* include polysaccharides, tannins, vitamin C, enzymes, resin, mineral salts, organic acids (phenolic, oleic, cerotic, linolic, palmitic, and caffeic acids), thirteen polyacetylene compounds, germacrene, methyl p-hydroxycinnamate, vanillin, and other components. Cichoric acid, most highly concentrated in the fresh flowers and roots, is thought to be involved in immunostimulatory action (Bauer, Remiger, and Wagner 1988a). Cichoric acid is also found in lower concentrations in *E. pallida* and *E. angustifolia.*

Bauer and Foster (1989) reported on the analysis of *E. simulata* and *E. paradoxa* roots, both endemic species from the Ozark Plateau. *Echinacea paradoxa's* lipophilic constituents were found to be nearly identical with the ketoalkene and -alkynes of *E. pallida.* *Echinacea paradoxa* also contained the alkamides. *Echinacea simulata* was shown to have similar alkamides to those found in *E. angustifolia.* In hydrophylic fractions, echinacoside was the primary component. Concentrations in *E. paradoxa* and *E. simulata* were comparable to those from *E. pallida* and *E. angustifolia.* In a recent study, Bauer, Remiger, and Alstat (1990) reported on the presence of alkamides and caffeic acid derivatives in the roots of the endangered species *E. tennesseensis.* Eight alkamides previously found in *E. angustifolia* were found. These were isobutylamides. Cynarine, also found in *E. angustifolia,* was discovered in *E. tennesseensis.* In short, the chemistry of *E. tennesseensis* was found to be very similar to *E. angustifolia.* However, it was surprising that the glycoside echinacoside was not found in *E. tennesseensis*.

Complete reviews of the history of chemical discovery in Echinacea and contemporary research can be found in Hobbs (1989) and the various papers of Bauer, Proksch, Wagner and their coworkers at the University of Munich.

Phytochemical studies of the remaining species of the genus are currently underway. It should be noted as well that a number of the chemical studies done on *E. angustifolia* and *E. purpurea* have been conducted on samples provided by the commercial herb market. Without an herbarium sheet (pressed plant specimen) or other scientifically verifiable specimen of the source plant, it is possible that some studies have inadvertently been conducted with *E. pallida, E. simulata, E. atrorubens,* or *E. paradoxa,* all of which are known to have entered the botanical trade in recent years.

Unfortunately, the exact identification of species, misidentification of specimens, a lack of voucher specimens for many chemical studies, and great variation in different lots of plant material, make many early chemical studies unreliable. It is now known that different Echinacea species have differing chemical compositions. Recent and repeated studies by Bauer and coworkers provide chromatographic fingerprints of various Echinacea species.

Future chemical and pharmacological studies should include chromatographic fingerprints of the commercial preparations or laboratory-prepared extracts under study, along with herbarium voucher specimens of plant materials used in experimentation. These can serve as references for verifying plant identity. Comparisons of the action of different species or forms of preparation, along with the detection of adulterants, can only be done if proper reference samples clearly establish identity and are available for inspection.

Proper identity involves not only chemistry, but also the skills of the field botanist and taxonomist. The two chapters to follow deal with Echinacea's botanical identity and distribution, as well as the history and evolution of botanical names that refer to the nine species we call Echinacea.

11

The Evolution of a Name: Wanderings in Taxonomic History

What's in a Name?

Botanical or scientific names are reference points, symbols for an individual plant. They are a common language used by botanists, horticulturists, herbalists, and plant enthusiasts.

Many botanical or Latin names also serve as common plant names, such as Sassafras, Forsythia, Gardenia, and Phlox. Echinacea is another example. As previously mentioned, the name is derived from a Greek word root *echinos* (denoting hedgehog or sea urchin), that refers to the sharp spiny projections on the cone-shaped seed heads.

Botanical names provide a simple, universal means to distinguish one plant from another. Based on the sum of their similarities and differences, botanists classify plants into various groupings. As an academic discipline, the study of plant classification principles and practices is known as taxonomy. Taxonomy is the starting point from which we may begin to document the human relationship to plants. Taxonomic history gives us a glimpse into the discovery of plants and their naming. After all, as John Hill said in his *Family Herbal* (1812), "it is in vain that we know betony is good for headaches or self-heal for wounds unless we can distinguish betony and self-heal from one another" (Foster 1984).

Echinacea: The Genus

Echinacea purpurea was the first Echinacea species described by botanists. Linnaeus described it in *Species Plantarum* (1753), calling it *Rudbeckia purpurea*, named in honor of a Swedish botanist, Olaf Rudbec. Linnaeus based his description on earlier published references, including L. Plunkenett (1696), who called it *Chrysanthemum americanum*, and Morrison, who in 1699 published the name *Drancunculus virginianus latifolius* (McGregor, 1968a). In 1790, N. J. de Necker published the name *Brauneria* in his *Elementa Botanica* in honor of an early eighteenth century German herbalist, Jacob Brauner. The generic name *Echinacea* was not published until four years later (1794) by Conrad Moench.

According to the International Code of Botanical Nomenclature —the rules botanists follow in naming plants—the first validly published name has "priority." It was recognized that Linnaeus's *Rudbeckia purpurea* belonged to a genus separate from *Rudbeckia*, and since *Brauneria* was the oldest generic name for the plant, it would seem to be the obvious choice for the genus name. However, many botanists disregarded Necker's *Brauneria* because he failed to describe a species (as the term is understood today) and did not adequately distinguish the differences between Linnaeus's *Rudbeckia* and his *Brauneria*. In his plant classification efforts, Necker used the terms *"species naturalis"* rather than the term genus, and used the term *"genera"* in reference to what are now known as plant families. The problem of Necker's *Brauneria* was solved in 1959 at the International Botanical Congress in Montreal, where it was decided that the names of Necker's *species naturalis* (including *Brauneria)* were invalid. Therefore, the name *Echinacea* became the undisputed choice for the genus name.

The genus had also been called *Bobartia* by J. Petiver in 1704. Constantine Samuel Rafinesque renamed the genus *Helichroa* in an 1825 work. He uses that name in the second volume of his *Medical Flora* (1830). Rafinesque's medicinal references to *E. purpurea* are seldom cited in historical treatments of *Echinacea* given the fact that he had obscured the identity of the plant with one of his infamous, erratic generic names.

Evolution of Species Names

Echinacea angustifolia DC was first described and named in 1836 by Augustin Pyramus DeCandolle. Heller (1900) listed it as *Brauneria angustifolia*. It was variously known to botanists as *Brauneria angustifolia* and *E. angustifolia,* until the generic problem was finally resolved in 1959. Arthur Cronquist (Hitchcock and Cronquist 1955) reduced *E. angustifolia* to a variety of *E. pallida* [*E. pallida* var. *angustifolia* (DC) Cronquist]. Hitchcock and Cronquist retain that classification in the 1976 edition of the *Flora of the Pacific Northwest.* In *Vascular Flora of the Southeastern States* vol. 1 (1980), Cronquist persists in treating *E. angustifolia* as a variety of *E. pallida.*

William J. Dress (1961, p. 77) treats *E. angustifolia* and *E. pallida* as separate entities. "The characters that distinguish the two taxa are not many nor great, and there is little to choose between considering them distinct species or two varieties of one; my own inclination is to maintain them as separate though closely related species."

In *The Taxonomy of the Genus Echinacea,* Ronald L. McGregor (1968a) recognized *E. pallida* and *E. angustifolia* as distinct species. McGregor also recognized two varieties of *E. angustifolia,* naming *E. angustifolia* DC var. *strigosa* McGregor (McGregor 1968b).

Echinacea atrorubens (Nutt.) Nutt. was first described and named *Rudbeckia purpurea* by the famous British-American naturalist, Thomas Nuttall, in 1834. Nuttall transferred the species to *Echinacea* in 1841. Nuttall collected it "in the plains of Arkansas, and also in Georgia, from whence I have received roots from my indefatigable friend, Dr. T. J. Wray" (Nuttall 1934, p. 80). Dr. Wray's material from Georgia was likely another taxon, perhaps *E. laevigata.* Nuttall describes the new plant as a "species closely related to *R. purpurea* and *R. pallida,* but perfectly distinct in its singular smoothness, very narrow entire leaves, and *dark red* rays, which are very showy from the intensity of their color."

Boynton and Beadle (1901) transferred *E. atrorubens* to *Brauneria atrorubens.* Errors in interpretations of this and other taxa placed under *E. atrorubens* by various nineteenth-century authors are examined and corrected by Boynton and Beadle. However in their treatment of the genus in Small's *Flora of the Southeastern United States* (1903, pp. 1261–1262) they further complicate the matter by including *E. paradoxa* under *Brauneria atrorubens* with no mention of synonymy. The complex errors and misinterpretations persisted until they were unraveled by McGregor (1968a).

Echinacea laevigata **(Boynton and Beadle) Blake,** a rare Appalachian species, was first described and named *Brauneria laevigata* in 1903 by Boynton and Beadle (in Small, 1903). Blake (1929) renamed it *Echinacea laevigata,* the name recognized by McGregor in 1968a. In 1945, A. Cronquist reduced the species to a variety of *E. purpurea (E. purpurea* var. *laevigata),* based on his belief that the only distinguishing feature separating *E. laevigata* from *E. purpurea* was that the former was essentially glabrous (smooth). Cronquist was apparently unaware of other distinguishing features such as *E. laevigata's* fusiform (carrot-shaped) root, and the length of the awn of the pales, both providing further reasons to separate the two species. However, Cronquist (1980) treats *E. laevigata* as a distinct species.

McGregor (1968a, p. 130) writes: *"E. laevigata* is a clearly defined species, but closely related to *E. purpurea."*

Echinacea pallida **(Nutt.) Nutt.** Thomas Nuttall first named *Echinacea pallida Rudbeckia pallida.* It is a plant "greatly resembling *R. purpurea,* but with very long petiolated narrow and almost perfectly entire leaves; the peduncle, or part of the stem destitute of leaves, fourteen to sixteen inches long. The rays pale purple, or almost rose red. . . . Arkansas. Collected by myself and Dr. Pitcher" (Nuttall 1834, p. 77).

In 1841 Nuttall recognized it as *Echinacea pallida*. *E. pallida* was figured and erroneously described as *E. angustifolia* by Sir William Jackson Hooker in *Curtis's Botanical Magazine* (1861). In 1894 Britton transferred it to *Brauneria pallida*. Since the time that botanical names of Necker were invalidated, the plant has been known as *E. pallida*.

Echinacea paradoxa (Norton) Britton var. *paradoxa* was first described and named *Brauneria paradoxa* by Norton in 1902. Britton (1913) reclassified it as *E. paradoxa*. Cronquist (1945) reduced it to the varietal level, *E. atrorubens* var. *paradoxa*. This is an extension of the confusion surrounding the identity and range of *E. atrorubens* and the fact that Boynton and Beadle, in their treatment of the genus in Small (1903), treat *E. paradoxa* as *E. atrorubens*. The problem was further compounded by confusion in the identity of *Echinacea* specimens from the Arbuckle mountains of Oklahoma, which McGregor (1968b) described as a new taxon *E. paradoxa* var. *neglecta*. In his monograph on the genus, McGregor (1968a) recognized *E. paradoxa* as a distinct, clearly defined species.

Echinacea purpurea (L.) Moench, as mentioned previously, was named *Drancunculus virginianus latifolius* by Morison (1699). Plunkenett (1696) called it *Chrysanthemum americanum*. Based on these works Linnaeus (1753) named the plant *Rudbeckia purpurea*. Moench (1794) described and named the genus *Echinacea*, under which *E. purpurea* was placed.

John Lindley (1849) described a form of *E. purpurea* as "*E. intermedia*" differing from the typical species principally in having spreading (rather than drooping) ray flowers.

Echinacea purpurea or its forms have also been variously called *Rudbeckia hispida, Echinacea serotina (R. serotina), Echinacea speciosa,* and *Brauneria purpurea* (McGregor 1968a). *Echinacea serotina* differed in supposedly being more hispid or hirsute (hairy) than typical *Echinacea purpurea* (Nicholson 1885–86).

Steyermark (1938) described and named *Echinacea purpurea* var. *arkansana,* based primarily on the fact that it is smaller in all respects than typical *E. purpurea*, and blooms earlier (May to June). McGregor however, questioned its taxonomic validity based on the fact that typical *E. purpurea* transplanted into an open experimental garden developed the characteristics of var. *arkansana*. Plants of variety *arkansana* grown by McGregor in a wooded habitat were identical to typical *E. purpurea* in size and flowering time (McGregor 1968a). McGregor considers the varietal status invalid, treating it as an early season ecological form associated with an open habitat (Correll and Johnston 1970).

Echinacea sanguinea **Nutt.** was named by Nuttall in 1841. Its taxonomic position has remained relatively stable, though Fernald (1900) considered it synonymous with *E. pallida* and Sharp (1935) wrote that it was a synonym for *E. angustifolia*.

Echinacea simulata **McGregor** is very similar to *E. pallida* and was first described and named by McGregor (1968b, 1968c). McGregor's original name for the taxon was *Echinacea speciosa*, but that name was found to be a homonym, thus invalid. (*E. speciosa* was published in reference to *E. purpurea* in 1849.)

Echinacea tennesseensis **(Beadle) Small,** one of the first species to be named to the federal endangered species list, has been treated as a separate species, a variety of *E. angustifolia*, and Fernald (1900) merged it with *E. angustifolia*. Beadle (1898) first described the plant as a distinct taxon, calling it *Brauneria tennesseensis*. Fernald (1900) argued against Beadle's "*Brauneria tennesseensis*" as distinct from *E. angustifolia*. Blake (1929) reduced it to a variety of *E. angustifolia*, also cited by Sharp (1935). Small (1933) gave the plant its present name and taxonomic position. McGregor (1968a) again recognized it as a distinct species. Cronquist (1980) treats this taxon as "an eastern outlier of [*E. pallida*] var. *angustifolia.*" Observations of living specimens of *E. tennesseensis* and the closely related *E. angustifolia* var. *angustifolia* reveals distinct organisms deserving of species status.

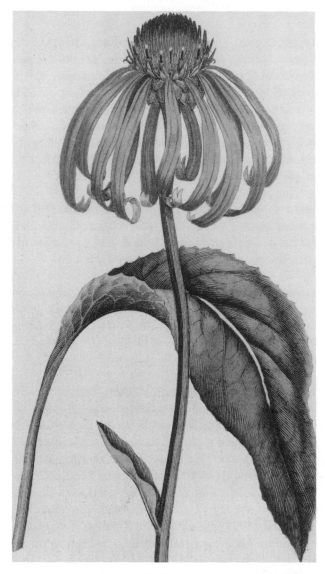

Echinacea purpurea *from Curtis's Botanical Magazine,*
Vol. 1, 1787, Plate no. 2. Courtesy of Hunt Institute for Botanical
Documentation, Carnegie Mellon University, Pittsburgh, PA.

12

Characteristics of the Genus Echinacea: The Botanist's View

The genus Echinacea is represented by nine species and two varieties indigenous to North America; the Echinaceas are perennial herbs with vertical or horizontal roots. The stems stand erect, singly or branched, and have rough, coarse hairs (hirsute), stiff bristly hairs (hispid), straight stiff hairs appressed toward the surface (strigose), and can be smooth, without hairs (glabrous), or the surface may be covered with a white substance that rubs off (glaucous).

On the lower part of the stem, the apparently alternate leaves have long stalks (petioles). Toward the top of the flower stalk, the leaves become progressively smaller and sessile (without petioles). The leaves are oval to lance shaped (ovate-lanceolate) or elliptical. Leaves are entire (without teeth) or coarsely toothed (in *E. purpurea* and *E. lacvigata),* and pubescent, or smooth.

The solitary flower head sits atop a long flower stalk (peduncle). The involucre—a set of leaflike structures (bracts)— encircles the stem directly below the flower head. The individual bracts are lance shaped. In the aster family (Compositae or Asteraceae) the bracts of the involucre are known as phyllaries. In Echinacea, the phyllaries are imbricate (overlapping) in a series of two or more. Closely studying an Echinacea flower will soon reveal that the phyllaries transform into pales as they move from the involucre to the flowers themselves. The pales are chaffy scales found just below (substending) the fruit of many Compositae. In Echinacea, the pales extend slightly beyond the corolla of each disk flower. They appear to be folded together lengthwise (conduplicate), and end in sharp, blunt, or slightly curved points. Once the flower head is dry, the pales remain intact, and form the chief feature of the dried flower. It is these spiny pales that prompt the name Echinacea (derived from the Greek *echinos,* meaning sea urchin or hedgehog).

The showy ray flowers surrounding each flower head are sterile. The long straplike ligules (ray flowers) have two or three slight or pronounced teeth at the ends. The ligules are white, pink, rose, purple, or even yellow in the case of *E. paradoxa* var. *paradoxa.* The fertile disk flowers are red-brown to green in color and inconspicuous compared to the ray flowers or even the pales, which are often tipped bright orange in *E. purpurea.* The corolla tubes of the disk flowers are cylindrical and five lobed. There are five stamens. The pollen is yellow or white. The small, one-seeded fruits (achenes) are four sided and have slight teeth at each corner of the crown.

The roots are taproots or fibrous (as in *E. purpurea).* The root has a sweetish taste at first, which upon prolonged chewing is acrid, tingling, and numbing, producing a numbing like that of clove oil, though without being hot or burning. This numbing effect is most pronounced in *E. angustifolia.* Echinacea root's numbing sensation has also been likened to aconite and cocaine, as well as to the prickly sensation of prickly ash *(Zanthoxylum).* The dried root is gray-brown or red brown, wrinkled and twisted lengthwise, often in a spiral. The root varies in size from that of a pencil to a large finger. The inner woody portion of the root, when cut transversely, exhibits yellow medullary rays separated by greenish gray fibers.

13

The Species: Identification and Distribution

The Common and Well-known Echinaceas

Echinacea angustifolia has simple or sometimes branched stems growing from six to twenty inches high. The stems are sparsely to densely covered with rough pubescence or stiff bristly hairs, sometimes swollen at their bases. The leaves have an oblong lance shape, without teeth, and are dark green with three to five nerves running the length of the blade. The ray flowers are mostly spreading (as opposed to drooping as in *E. pallida)* and are very short (¾ to 1⅜ inches long). The ray flowers are shorter than or as wide as the width of the disk.

Echinacea angustifolia is found on barrens and dry prairies from Minnesota to Texas, in western Oklahoma, Kansas, Nebraska, and Iowa, the Dakotas, eastern Colorado, Wyoming, and Montana, and extreme southern Saskatchewan and Manitoba.

McGregor's *E. angustifolia* var. *strigosa* is somewhat smaller, more branched, has strigose rather than tu-

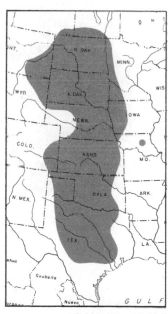

Echinacea angustifolia

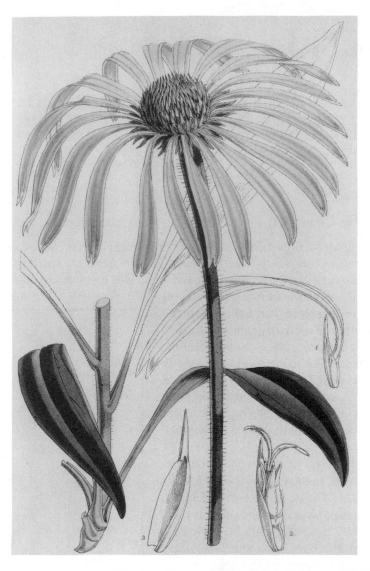

*Echinacea pallida from Curtis's Botanical Magazine, Vol. 87,
1861, Plate no. 5281 (erroneously labled Echinacea angustifolia).
Courtesy of Hunt Institute for Botanical Documentation, Carnegie
Mellon University, Pittsburgh, PA.*

berculate-hirsute or hispid hairs, and has stems that tend to curve alternately in opposite directions. Upon drying, the lower part of the stem is nearly smooth (glabrous) and green.

It has a narrow range, from north central Texas (east of the Panhandle) through central Oklahoma. Historically, significant amounts of root material labeled *E. angustifolia* on the American herb market are suspected to be *E. pallida.*

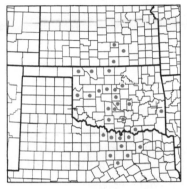

Echinacea angustifolia *var.* strigosa

Echinacea pallida is quite similar to *E. angustifolia,* though it is stouter and taller, growing to a height of thirty-nine inches. The narrow ray flowers are strongly reflexed—drooping and curving toward the stem —and quite long (1½ to 3½ inches long). The pales of the flower head tend to be longer than those of *E. angustifolia.*

Echinacea pallida is the only Echinacea with white pollen. The ray flowers are pale white to deep purple. Flowers tend to be lighter in color in the southern part of its range, becoming darker and richer in color in northern populations. It flowers from early June through July.

Echinacea pallida has a more eastern and broader range than *E. angustifolia,* occurring in open

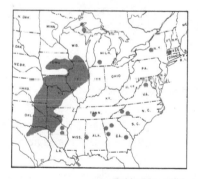

Echinacea pallida

woods, glades, and rocky prairies from northeast Texas, eastern Oklahoma, and Kansas north to Iowa and Wisconsin, and east to Indiana. Eastward to Pennsylvania and Georgia, sparse populations are considered to have been introduced or locally established. It is relatively unusual east of Illinois.

Echinacea purpurea grows from two to five feet tall, often branching toward the top. The leaves have coarse pubescence. Lowermost leaves are oval to broadly lance shaped and coarsely toothed with irregular teeth. This is a key characteristic for distinguishing this species from the other common Echinaceas. The flower heads are large and colorful (up to seven inches across in some cultivated varieties, known as "cultivars"). The ray flowers are rose to deep purple, rarely white. The pales are often tipped bright orange, distinguishing this Echinacea from others at a quick glance. This is a good characteristic to remember if you're like me and like to identify plants while driving down the highway. It flowers from June through October.

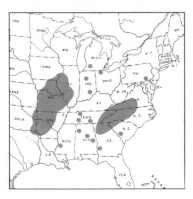
Echinacea purpurea

Echinacea purpurea is the most widely distributed, though not the most common species of Echinacea. It grows in open woods, prairies, and thickets from Louisiana, the northeastern tip of Texas, and eastern Oklahoma north through Ohio, Michigan, and eastward.

Echinacea purpurea is often grown as an ornamental perennial. It is by far the best-known Echinacea species in cultivation. Some plant sellers and seedsmen persist in selling it under the name *Rudbeckia purpurea.* Obsolete since 1841, the use of that name should be discouraged. There are several cultivars available including 'The King,' with bright crimson rays; 'Bright Star,' with rosy red rays and a maroon center; 'Sombrero,' sporting crimson-purple rays; and 'New Colewall Strain,' an English cultivar with heads six to seven inches wide and a greenish-bronze center. Though 'New Colewall Strain,' and another compact purple-red cultivar named 'Robert Bloom' are listed in gardening books, I have yet to see them in a catalog. German cultivars with carmine red rays and large heads include 'Abendsonne,' 'Auslese,' and 'Leuchtstern.'

'Bressingham Hybrid' has a dark cone with bright rose ray florets. 'Earliest of All,' another English cultivar, has pink-purple ray flowers.

White-flowered cultivars with green disks and orange pales include 'Alba,' 'White Prince,' 'White King,' and 'White Lustre.' McGregor (1968a) reports that all of these variations have been found in the wild. In 1987 Thompson & Morgan introduced a new white-flowered dwarf cultivar named 'White Swan.' A recent cultivar from the German firm Klaus Jelitto, called 'Magnus,' sports white, spreading blooms.

Breeders at German firms have strived to develop cultivars with spreading (as opposed to drooping) petals in response to a notion of German plant buyers. Apparently German consumers believe that those specimens with drooping petals are wilted or diseased.

Echinacea purpurea has been cultivated for at least two hundred years. It was introduced into English gardens at an early date. William Townsend Aiton noted that the plant had been introduced "before 1699, by the Rev. John Banister" (Ewan and Ewan 1970). By the time that the second volume of W. P. C. Barton's *A Flora of North America* was published in 1822, *E. purpurea* was recognized as "one of the most showy of our native plants, and has long been cultivated in gardens in this country and Europe. It is a hardy plant, enduring the cold of our climate very well, and improving in vigour by cultivation" (pp. 85–86).

The second plate published in *Curtis's Botanical Magazine* (1787), perhaps the best known periodical of botanical illustrations, was of *E. purpurea*.

Not withstanding it is a native of the warm climates of Carolina and Virginia, it succeeds very well with us in an open border; but as Mr. Miller very justly observes, it will always be prudent to shelter two or three plants under a common hot-bed frame in winters, those in the open air are sometimes killed. It flowers in July. As it rarely ripens its seeds with us, the only mode of propagating it, is by parting the root; but in that way the plant does not admit of much increase (Curtis 1787, vol. 1, pl. 2).

The second plate is captioned "Botanic Garden, Lambeth Marsh 1786." Later, Curtis transformed this, his personal garden, into the London Botanic Garden, opening it to the public in January 1779. One major question arises from the description above. Why did such a hardy plant, which seeds even in central Maine, need greenhouse protection during the winter months in southern England? The answer may lie in the fact that Curtis mentions its native home as "Carolina and Virginia." Perhaps the plant depicted as plate 2 in the first issue of Curtis's *Botanical Magazine,* may instead have been *E. laevigata*—a plant native, though rare, in Virginia and the Carolinas, and perhaps not hardy further north. If one studies the plate carefully, it appears that the awns of the pales are short, extending from near the crown of the pales. This is an important characteristic separating *E. laevigata* from *E. purpurea,* which has relatively long awns (half the length of the pale). Fernald (1950) included incurved tips of the pales in his description of *E. laevigata.* The tips of the pales depicted in the Curtis plate are obviously incurved. The long recurved petals depicted in the plate are more typical to *E. laevigata* than *E. purpurea.*

Lesser Known and Unusual Species

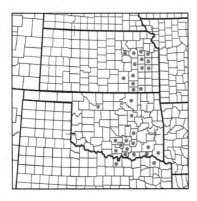

Echinacea atrorubens

Echinacea atrorubens, a rare endemic of the eastern edge of Oklahoma and Kansas, has been threatened in recent years from injudicious collecting. It grows to three feet tall and has light green, glabrous stems. Lower leaves and stems may have some pubescence. *Echinacea atrorubens* has short ray flowers like *E. angustifolia,* but they are so dramatically reflexed as to touch the flower stalks. The rays are dark purple, rarely pink or white.

It grows on prairies in a very narrow range, from Houston, Texas, to Ardmore, Oklahoma, and north to the Topeka, Kansas, area.

Echinacea paradoxa var. *paradoxa* is the most unusual "purple coneflower," given the paradox that its ray flowers are yellow. It grows to four feet in height, and like *E. atrorubens,* has light green stems and leaves. The plant is smooth or only slightly hairy. The disk is usually dark brown. The ray flowers are yellow, rarely white or peach (I have seen one specimen with orange ray

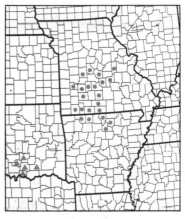

● Echinacea paradoxa
▲ Echinacea paradoxa var. neglecta

flowers, perhaps a hybrid with *E. simulata). Echinacea paradoxa* flowers appear in mid to late May or early June and last into July, though I have seen individuals bloom as early as 30 March.

It grows on glades, bald knobs, in open woods, and rocky prairies. It is endemic to the south central and western Arkansas Ozarks and central, southern, and western Missouri counties. It is known from at least seventeen Missouri counties and five Arkansas counties.

Echinacea paradoxa var. *neglecta,* endemic to the Arbuckle Mountains of Oklahoma, is distinguished by its rose, purple, or white ray flowers.

Echinacea sanguinea has the southernmost distribution of the genus, occurring in southwest Arkansas, southeastern Oklahoma, western Louisiana, and eastern Texas. It grows in open sandy fields and open pine woods. The flower head is nearly hemispherical: it

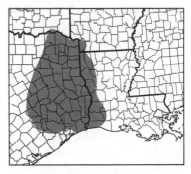

Echinacea sanguinea

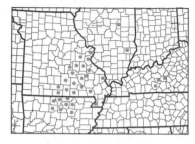

Echinacea simulata

has slender stems and narrow dark red, rarely white, ray flowers. The pollen is yellow. The basal leaves are elliptical.

Echinacea simulata is very similar to *E. pallida,* but is distinguished by its yellow rather than white pollen, which is smaller than that of *E. pallida.* According to McGregor (1968a), *E. pallida* is a polyploid with n=22, while *E. simulata* has n=11. It occurs in north central Arkansas, eastern and south central Missouri, southwestern Illinois, and west central Kentucky.

Endangered Species

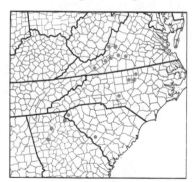

Echinacea laevigata

Echinacea laevigata is very similar to *E. purpurea,* but is nearly glabrous, has narrower leaves, is rarely branched, and has a bifid (forked) tap root. The ray flowers are somewhat longer and narrower than those of *E. purpurea.* The bristles (awn) of the pales are a quarter as long as the main part of the pale and have curved tips, (the awn of the chaff in *E. purpurea* is half as long as the body). It has been found in Pennsylvania, Virginia, the Carolinas, Georgia, and is reported from northeastern Alabama. The plant forms small stands in open woods or grassy glades. This species is currently under review by the United States Fish and Wildlife Service for endangered species status. Only fifteen populations are known.

Echinacea tennesseensis, known from five natural populations in dry, gravel cedar barrens of central Tennessee, is very rare. On 6 June 1979, the United States Fish and Wildlife Service officially listed it as an endangered species. Its clos-

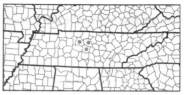

Echinacea tennesseensis

est relative is *E. angustifolia* var. *angustifolia,* though it is considered specifically distinct. It is somewhat larger in habit than *E. angustifolia,* has more leafy stems, softer pubescence, and smaller pollen grains. Unlike other Echinacea species, *E. tennesseensis,* is characterized by upturned rather than drooping ray flowers. Flowering begins as early as mid May, peaks in June and July, and may last as late as October.

The species was collected as early as 1878 by Dr. A. Gattinger in Rutherford County, Tennessee. Gattinger apparently considered it to be *E. angustifolia.* However, the type specimen for this taxon was not collected until 19 August 1897 by H. G. Eggert.

It is very possible that some populations known in the late nineteenth century were extirpated by root diggers seeking *E. angustifolia.* In *Medicinal Plants of Tennessee* (1894), Dr. A. Gattinger lists *E. angustifolia* as a medicinal plant of the state occurring "in cedar glades, rather infrequent."

The species was thought to be very rare or possibly extinct by McGregor (1968a), but in that same year it was rediscovered in an open cedar glade in central Tennessee. A team of five Tennessee botanists have developed a recovery plan for this species with the ultimate aim of removing it from the endangered species list. The plan includes propagating the species from seeds collected at wild populations or from cultivated specimens. In recent years, seeds have been available through the American Rock Garden Society's seed exchange program. Limited numbers of plants have been made available through Cheekwood Botanical Gardens in Nashville, the Endangered Species Plant Exchange, and three commercial nurseries licensed to sell the plant (see Plant and Seed Sources).

14

The Need for Conservation: Is Time Running Short?

The historical harvesting of Echinacea, for both European and American markets, has had a profound impact on wild populations of Echinacea. That impact has grown in severity in contemporary times, as harvesting of the wild plant has only intensified.

Two generations ago, Professor L. E. Sayre (1897, 1898, 1903, 1904, 1915, 1916) warned of pressure on wild populations in Kansas. "For the past ten years the demand for the root of this plant [*Echinacea angustifolia* and *E. pallida*] has been gradually increasing until now it is so great that there seems to be a danger of the extermination of the plant. . . . About a month ago we had a call from an agent of an Eastern house for the purchase of 40,000 pounds and from another of 20,000 pounds; other parties have written asking for smaller lots of two or three hundred pounds each" (1904, p. 5).

The demand prompted Sayre to write to Rodney True of USDA's Bureau of Plant Industry, "asking that something be done toward the protection of the plant, or measures be taken for its cultivation." True apparently agreed to study cultivation of the plant, though little seems to have come of this work (1904, p. 5).

Sayre noted that at the 1903 meeting of the Kansas Academy of Sciences, one person who attended stated that 200,000 pounds of the root had been collected from Rooks County, Kansas, the previous year. Kindscher (1989) states that about 2 million roots must have been harvested in that year alone, given the fact that eight to ten (or more) dried roots are required for just one pound.

Five years ago there was a report of an herb buyer in Missouri who supposedly ships 30,000 pounds of wild Echinacea roots and tops to the European market each year. That figure is now far greater. Dr. James H. Wilson, former Endangered Species Coordinator, Missouri Department of Conservation, says "We are seeing a substantial decrease in coneflowers along Missouri roadsides in recent years" (personal communication, 14 March 1984).

Missouri law requires that a person harvesting any plant material for commercial use must have permission of the land owner to do so. Along roadside right-of-ways, the owner is the State of Missouri. The increased coneflower harvest has prompted Missouri Department of Conservation officials to begin to monitor populations of the plant on state-owned lands and to begin prosecuting persons illegally harvesting plants.

McGregor (1968a) reported that research developed a sudden demand for the root in 1965, resulting in the harvest of 25,000 pounds of the dried root in one year. *Echinacea pallida* was apparently the most desired species at the time, though *E. angustifolia* was harvested as well. Since the last edition of this book was published in late 1985, the stress on wild populations has become greater.

More recently, (1987) Ronald McGregor, Director Emeritus of the Herbarium at the University of Kansas and the leading authority on the botany of Echinacea, explains that the problem has become more acute.

Over the past 25 years, but especially within the last five, I have noted a rather drastic decline in Kansas populations of *Echinacea pallida*. Last summer I observed a crew of six persons with a one-and-a-half ton truck filled with bags of roots and was told that it was their eleventh load so far in the season, and that was around the first of June.

The digging of *Echinacea angustifolia* is much less extensive in Kansas largely because the roots are smaller and harder to dig. If the price increases, however, it is certain populations of *Echinacea angustifolia* will decline.

In my opinion we will have a real problem on our hands with native populations before we are able to develop some sort of control. Because populations are still rather frequent it is difficult to create much interest on the part of those in a position to act. Though I carefully explain the drastic decline in populations in recent years, I receive little attention. If *Echinacea* had a little fur and cute little black eyes, one could elicit a little attention! In Kansas, only the Fish and Game Commission has any control over endangered and threatened species but they will only consider animals. We indeed have a hard row to hoe (personal communication, 24 March 1987).

Similar pressures on Echinacea populations are occurring in Oklahoma, Arkansas, Kansas, Nebraska, Texas, the Dakotas, and other states in which Echinacea root is dug from the wild. The need for commercial cultivation of *E. angustifolia* and *E. pallida* becomes obvious.

Unfortunately, a number of the endemic and more unusual Echinacea species are entering commercial lots, dug by unwitting harvesters. In the Ozarks, this author has observed *E. simulata,* harvested by the truck load. Roadside populations have decreased dramatically in south central Missouri. The plant is much less common in northern Arkansas. Commercial harvest of this species from the wild cannot be sustained. If harvested at current levels over the next ten years, its fate will be extinction.

In the winter of 1987, officials at Missouri's Ha Ha Tonka State Park reported the theft of nearly 7,000 yellow coneflowers *(E. paradoxa)* from a glade at the park. This species is known only from seventeen Missouri counties and five Arkansas counties. Commercial harvest of this plant should be prohibited.

The endemic *E. atrorubens* is also being harvested and thrown into mixed lots of material sold as *"E. angustifolia."* Dr. McGregor has observed its decline. "Last season I failed to locate colonies of *E. atrorubens* in the few prairies where I knew it once occurred. I was told by landowners that the plants had been dug by diggers without permission" (personal communication, 7 April 1987).

The federally listed endangered species, *E. tennesseensis,* was likely harvested as a medicinal plant in the late nineteenth century. Gattinger (1894) lists it (as *E. angustifolia*) among the medicinal plants of Tennessee, describing its occurrence in the habitat of the Tennessee Coneflower. Now known from only five natural populations, one person could wipe this species out in a day's digging. The Appalachian species, *E. laevigata,* known only from fifteen populations, many along roadsides or power lines, is threatened. Now under review for endangered species status, it should be carefully preserved.

Cultivation of all of these species should be pursued in earnest. *E. tennesseensis* and *E. laevigata* are relatively easy to grow. Vigorous propagation efforts must be funded by federal, state or private sources. The two major wild populations of *E. tennesseensis* remain on unprotected private land, threatened by residential encroachment. At least two known populations have already been destroyed. The Nature Conservancy of Tennessee has been unsuccessful in raising the money necessary to purchase the major populations.

To sell a federally listed endangered species one must have a license from the United States Fish and Wildlife Service. Several nurseries now have licenses to sell the Tennessee Coneflower. Some, however, sell other species of Echinacea as well, and cannot guarantee that Tennessee Coneflower seeds will come true to form. Echinaceas hybridize readily. Those licensed to propagate *E. tennesseensis* should, in my opinion, not grow other species of Echinacea in close proximity. The genetic integrity of endangered species must be protected, as well as their habitats.

Propagation and cultivation of Echinacea species is the solution to the conservation problem. Commercial cultivation of the relatively easily grown *E. purpurea* is well under way, as is cultivation of *E. pallida.* The more desirable, higher-priced, and difficult to cultivate *E. angustifolia* has yet to be established as a commercial crop on any scale. Through concerted effort and cooperation among conservationists, entrepreners, and researchers, it will be possible to establish Echinacea as a valued cultivated herb.

 Plant and Seed Sources

Abundant Life Seed Foundation
P.O. Box 772
Port Townsend, WA 98368
> *E. angustifolia, E. purpurea* seed, retail/wholesale.

Elixir Farm Botanicals
General Delivery
Brixey, MO 65618
> *E. angustifolia, E. pallida, E. paradoxa, E. purpurea* seed,
> retail/wholesale.

HG German Seeds
Box 398
201 West Main Street
Smethport, PA 16749
> *E. purpurea* seed, wholesale.

Missouri Wildflowers Nursery
Rt. 2, Box 373
Jefferson City, MO 65109
> *E. pallida, E. paradoxa, E. purpurea* seeds and plants, retail.

Native Gardens
Rt. 1, Box 494
Greenback, TN 37742
> *E. paradoxa, E. purpurea, E. tennesseensis** plants, retail.

Natural Gardens
4804 Shell Lane
Knoxville, TN 37918
> *E. purpurea, E. tennesseensis** plants.

---

* Licensed to sell *E. tennesseensis* under permit issued by the United States Fish & Wildlife Service.

Otto Richter & Sons
Goodwood
Ontario, Canada LOC 1A0
  E. angustifolia, and *E. purpurea* seed, retail/wholesale.

Prairie Nursery
P.O. Box 365
Westfield, WI 53964
  E. pallida and *E. purpurea* seed and plants, retail/wholesale.

Prairie Moon Nursery
Rt. 3, Box 163
Winona, MN 55987
  E. angustifolia, E. pallida, and *E. purpurea* seed and plants,
  retail/wholesale.

Prairie Ridge Nursery
RR 2, 9738 Oberland Rd.
Mt. Horeb, WI 53572-2832
  E. pallida, E. purpurea seed and plants, retail/wholesale.

Sunlight Gardens
Rt. 1, Box 600-A
Hillvale Rd.
Andersonville, TN 37705
  *E. pallida, E. purpurea, E. tennesseensis** plants, retail.

We-Du Nurseries
Rt. 5, Box 724
Marion, NC 28752
  E. paradoxa, E. purpurea plants, retail.

Please note, many of these businesses charge for their catalog. Send
$1.00 or a postcard to inquire about the charge. Numerous additional
sources of perennial seeds and plants also offer *E. purpurea* and its
cultivars.

---

* Licensed to sell *E. tennesseensis* under permit issued by the United States
Fish & Wildlife Service.

Bibliography

Albus, G. and H. Hering.1941. *Med. Klinik* 37:276.

Alken, C.E. 1951. *Med. Klinik* 46(44):1145–49.

Am. Pharm. Assn. 1918. *The national formulary*. 4th ed. Philadelphia.

Arnulphy, B.S. 1926. *Allg. Hom-Ztg.* 174:75.

Auster, F. and J. Schäfer. 1957. *Echinacea angustifolia*. D. C. Leipzig: Thieme.

Baetgen, D. 1964. *Med. Mschr.* 18(3):129–31.

———. 1984. *Therapiewoche* 34(36):5115–19.

———. 1988. *TW Pädiatrie* 1(1):66–70.

Bailey, L.H. 1924. *Manual of cultivated plants*. New York: Macmillan.

Bailey, L.H. and Ethel Zoe Bailey. 1976. *Hortus third*. New York: Macmillan.

Bame, G.A. 1984. Biological and chemical analysis of *Echinacea pallida* (Nutt.) Nutt. Unpub. Master's thesis, South Sakota State University.

Barone, J. 1988. An herb called Echinacea. *American Health* (Nov.):124–25.

Barton, W.P.C. 1821–1823. *A flora of North America*. 3 vols. Philadelphia: H.C. Carey & I. Lea.

Baskin, J.M. and C. C. Baskin. 1982. Effects of vernalization and photoperiod on flowering in *Echinacea tennesseensis*, an endangered species. *J. Tenn. Acad. Sci.* 57(2):53–56.

Bauer, K. M. 1957. *Medizinishe* (1957):1863.

———. 1958. *Medizinishe* (1958):1921.

Bauer, R. and S. Foster. 1989. HPLC analysis of *Echinacea simulata* and *E. paradoxa* roots. *Planta Medica* 55:637.

Bauer, R., I. A. Khan, and H. Wagner. 1986. *Deutsche Apotheker Zeitung* 126:1065–70.

———. 1987. *Deutsche Apotheker Zeitung* 127:1325–30.

———. 1988. TLC and HPLC analysis of *Echinacea pallida* and *E. angustifolia* roots. *Planta Medica* 54:426–30.

Bauer, R., I. Khan, K. Jurcic and H. Wagner. 1986. Immunologically active sesquiterpene esters from *Parthenium integrifolium* and adulterant of

Echinacea purpurea. Poster presented at Biologically Active Natural Products Symposium Phytochemical Society of Europe, 3–5 Sept. 1986, Lausanne, Switzerland.

Bauer, R. I. Khan, H. Lotter, and H. Wagner.1985a. New constituents of *Echinacea purpurea.* Paper presented at International Research Congress on Natural Products, 7–12 July, 1985, at the University of North Carolina, Chapel Hill.

————. 1985b. Structure and stereochemistry of new sesquiterpene esters from *Echinacea purpurea* (L.) Moench. *Helv. Chim. Acta* 68:2355–58.

Bauer, R. I. Khan, V. Wary, and H. Wagner. 1987. Two acetylenic compounds from *Echinacea pallida* roots. *Phytochemistry* 26(4):1198–1200.

Bauer, R., K. Jurcic, J. Puhlmann and H. Wagner. 1988. *Arzneimittel Forschung* 38(1):276–81.

Bauer, R. and P. Remiger. 1989a. *Arch. Pharm.* (Weinheim) 322:324.

Bauer, R. and P. Remiger. 1989b. TLC and HPLC analysis of alkamides in *Echinacea* drugs. *Planta Medica* 55:367–71.

Bauer, R., P. Remiger and E. Alstat. 1990. Alkamides and caffeic acid derivatives from the roots of *Echinacea tennesseensis.* Poster presented at Biology and Chemistry of Active Natural Substances Symposium, 17–22 July, 1990. Bonn, West Germany

Bauer, R., P. Remiger and H. Wagner. 1988a. *Deutsche Apotheker Zeitung* 128(4):174–79.

————. 1988b. Alkamides from the roots of *Echinacea angustifolia. Phytochemistry* 27(7):2339–42.

————. 1989. Alkamides from the roots of *Echinacea angustifolia. Phytochemistry* 28(2):505–8.

Bauer, R., P. Remiger, K. Jurcic. and H. Wagner. 1989. *Zeitschrift für Phytotherapie* 10:43–48.

Bauer, R., P. Remiger, V. Wary, and H. Wagner. 1988. A germacrene alcohol from fresh aerial parts of *Echinacea purpurea. Planta medica* 54:478.

Bauer, R. and H. Wagner. 1987. Comments on the Echinacea problem. *Am. Herb Assn. Quart.* 5(3):4.

————. 1987. *Sci Pharm.* 55:159–61.

————. 1988a. *Zeitschrift für Phytotherapie* 9:151–59.

————. 1988b. Erratum: Echinacea-drogen—Who is who? *Zeitschrift für Phytotherapie* 9:191–92.

————. 1990. *Echinacea handbuch für ärtze, apotheker und andere naturwissenschaftler.* Stuttgart, W. Germany: Wissenschaftliche Verlagsgesellschaft mbH.

Beadle, C.D. 1898. Notes on the botany of the Southeastern United States, II. *Bot. Gaz.* 25:359–75.

Beal, J.M. 1921. Summary of the physiological report of Couch and Giltner. *Am. Jour. Pharm.* 93:229–32.

Becker, H. 1982. *Deutsche Apotheker Zeitung* 122(45):2320–23.

Becker, H., et. al. 1982. Structure of Echinacoside from *Echinacea angustifolia* Z. *Naturforsch Sect. C. Biosci.* 37(5–6):351–53.

Benigni, R., C. Capra, and P. E. Cattorini. 1962. Echinacea. *In. Piante medicinali. chimica, farmacologia e terapia.* Milan: Inverni & Della Betta.

Beringer, G. M. 1911. Fluid extract of Echinacea. *Am. Jour. Pharm.* 83:324.

Berkeley, E. and D.S. Berkeley. 1963. *John Clayton: pioneer of American botany.* Chapel Hill: University of North Carolina Press.

Berman, A. 1954. The impact of the nineteenth century botanico-medicial movement on American pharmacy and medicine. Unpublished doctoral dissertation, University of Wisconsin, Madison.

Beuscher, N., H. Beuscher, B. Otto, B. Schäffer. 1977. *Arzneimittel Forschung* 27:1655–60.

Beuscher, N, H. Beuscher, and B. Schäfer. 1978. *Arzneimittel Forschung* 28:2242–46.

Beuscher, N. 1980. *Arzneimittel Forschung* 30:821–25.

Bigelow, J.M. 1849. To the medical profession of Ohio. *Ohio Med. and Surg. Jour.* 2:97–143.

Birkenfeld, B. 1954. *Therapie Der Gegenwart* 93(11).

Bischoff, F. 1924. Oil of *Echinacea angustifolia*. *J. Am. Pharm. Assoc.* 13:898–902.

Blake, A.K. 1935. Viability and germination of seeds of prairie plants. *Ecol. Monogr.* 5:405–60.

Blake, S.F. 1929. New Asteraceae from the United States, Mexico, and Honduras. *Jour. Wash. Acad. Sci.* 19:273.

Blankenship, J.W.A. 1905. Native economic plants of Montana. *Montana Agri. Exp. Stn. Bulletin* 56:1–38.

Bohl, R. and T. Hermann. 1954. *Schweizerische Med. Wochenschrift* 84(15):421.

Bohlmann, F. and M. Grenz. 1966. Polyacetylene compounds 228. Biogenesis of polyanamides. *Chem. Ber.* 107(6):2120–22.

Bohlmann, F. and H. Hoffmann. 1983. Further amides from *Echinacea purpurea*. *Phytochemistry* 22(5):1173–75.

Bomme, U. 1986. *Merkblätter für Pflanzenbau.* Munich.

Bonadeo, I., G. Botazzi, and M. Lavazza. 1971. Echinacin B, an active polysaccharide from Echinacea. *Riv. Ital. Essenze, Profumi, Piante Offic., Armoi, Saponi, Cosmetici, Aerosol* 53(5):281–95.

Bonadeo, I. and M. Lavazza. 1972. Echinacina B: suo azione sui fibroblasti. *Riv. Ital. Essenze Profumi.* 54:195.

Boyce, S. R. 1893. *Echinacea angustifolia. Proc. Am. Pharm. Assn.* 79:479.

Boyd, L.J. 1928. Pharmacology of the homeopathic drugs. *J. Am. Inst. Homeopathy* 21:209–21.

Boynton, C.L. and C.D. Beadle. 1901. Notes on certain coneflowers. *Bilt Bot. Studies* 1:11–12.

_____. 1903. Brauneria. In J.K. Small, *Flora of the Southeastern United States.* pp. 1261–62. New York: J.K. Small.

British Herbal Medicine Association Scientific Committee.1979. *British herbal pharmacopeia.* West Yorks, England: British Herbal Medical Association.

_____. 1990. *British herbal pharmacopeia.* Dorset, England: British Herbal Medical Association.

Britton, N. L. 1894. *Mem. Torr. Bot. Club* 5:333 34.

Britton, N.L. and A. Brown. 1913. *Illustrated flora of the Northeastern United States and adjacent Canada.* 3 vols. 2nd. ed. New York: New York Botanical Garden.

Brandrup, W. 1969. Certain chapters of the *Homeopathic Pharmacopeia. Pharm. Ztg.* 81:548–49.

Broglie, M. 1954. *Dtsh. Med. Wschr.* (1954):769 & 816.

Büsing, K.H. 1952. Inhibition of hyaluronidase by Echinacin®. *Arzneimittel Forschung* 2:467–69.

_____. 1955. Hyaluronidase inhibition of some naturally occurring substances used in therapy. *Arzneimittel Forschung* 5:320–22.

_____. 1958. The effect of extracts from *Echinacea purpurea* on the properdin levels in rabbits. *Z. Immunitätsforsch. exper. Ther.* 115:169–76.

Büsing, K.H., and G. Thürigen. 1958. *Allerg. Asthma* 4:30–33.

Campbell, T.N. 1951. Medicinal plants used by the Choctaw, Chickasaw, and Creek Indians of the early nineteenth century. *Jour. Wash. Acad. Sci.* 41:285–90.

Carlson, G.A. and V.H. Jones. 1939. Some notes and uses of plants by the Comanche Indians. *Papers of the Michigan Academy of Sciences, Arts, and Letters* Vol. XXV. Ann Arbor: Univ. of Mich. Press.

Cassady, J.M., W.M. Baird, and C.J. Chang. 1990. Natural products as a source of potential cancer chemotherapeutic and chemopreventative agents. *Jour. Nat. Prod.* 53(1):23–41.

Caster, J.C. and G. A. Myers. 1987. A study of oleoresin canals in *Echinacea purpurea* (L.) Moench. *Proc. S. D. Acad. Sci.* 66:71–75.

Catesby, M. 1771. *The natural history of Carolina, Florida, and the Bahama Islands.* 2 vols. 3rd. ed. London.

Chapman, A.W. 1855. *Flora of the Southern States.* New York.

Cheminat, A., R. Zawatzky, H. Becker, and R. Broulliard. 1988. Caffeoyl conjugates from Echinacea species: structures and biological activity. *Phytochemistry* 27(9):2787–94.

Chone, B. 1965. *Arzneimittel Forschung* 19(11):611–12.

Chone, B. and G. Manidakis. 1969. *Dtsch. Med. Wschr.* 94(27):1406–10.

Christopher, J.R. 1976. *School of natural healing.* Provo, Utah: BiWorld.

Clapp, A. 1852. A report on medical botany. . . *Trans. of the AMA* 5:698–906.

Coeugniet, E. 1988. *Natura-Med.* 6:274–75.

Coeugniet, E. and E. Elek. 1987. Immunomodulation with *Viscum album* and *Echinacea purpurea* extracts. *Onkologie* 10(3):27–33.

Coeugniet, E. and R. Kühnast. 1986. *Therapiewoche* 36(33):3352–58.

Commission E. 1990. Draft monograph: Echinaceae herba (aerial parts of the coneflower). Berlin: BGA.

Cooke, M.P. 1979. Stereoselective synthesis of the proposed American coneflower juvenile hormone mimic. *J. Org. Chem.* 44(14):2461–68.

Correll, D.S. and M.C. Johnston. 1970. *Manual of the vascular plants of Texas.* Renner, Texas: Texas Research Foundation.

Couch, J.F. and L.T. Giltner. 1920. An experimental study of Echinacea therapy. *Journ. Agric. Res.* 20:63–84.

———. 1921. Echinacea—a reply to Dr. Beal. *Am. Jour. Pharm.* 93:234–39.

Coulter, H. L. 1973. *Divided legacy: a history of schism in medical thought.* Vol. III. Science and ethics in American medicine: 1800–1914. Washington, D.C.: McGrath Publishing Company.

Council on Pharmacy and Chemistry. 1909. Echinacea considered valueless. *JAMA* 53(22):1836.

Cronquist, A. 1945. Notes on the Compositae of the Northeastern United States. II Heliantheae and Helenieae. *Rhodora* 47:396–403.

———. 1980. *Vascular flora of the Southeastern United States.* Vol. 1. *Asteraceae.* Chapel Hill: Univ. of N.C. Press.

Croom, E.M. 1983. Documenting and evaluating herbal remedies. *Economic Botany* 37(1):13–27.

Curtis, W. 1787. *Rudbeckia purpurea.* Purple Rudbeckia. *Curtis's Botanical Magazine* Vol. 1, plate 2.

Cutler, S.H. 1930. The inorganic constituents of Echinacea. *J. Am. Pharm. Assoc.* 19:120–21.

———. 1931. Echinacea: a phytochemical study. *Bull. Univ. Wisc.*, Ser. No. 1787, Gen. Ser. No. 1571.

DeCandolle, A.P. and A. DeCandolle. 1836. *Prodromus systematis naturalis regni vegetabilis.* Vol. 5 p. 554–55. Paris.

Doesel, H. 1977. *Taegl. Praxis* 18:21–40.

Doetsch, H. 1985. *Kneipp-Physiotherapie* 5(1):14–17.

Dopp, W. et. al. 1950. Tuberculiostatic action of some plant extracts *in vitro Pharmazie* 5:603–4.

Dress, W.J. 1961. Notes on the cultivated Compositae 6. The coneflowers: *Dracopsis, Echinacea, Ratibida, Rudbeckia. Baileya* 9:67–83.

_____. 1983. Personal communication. 5 December.

Dudzus, G. 1951. *Tierärztl. Umschau* 9/10:172.

Duke, J.A. 1979. *Echinacea angustifolia.* Unpublished notes provided to the author by J.A. Duke.

_____. 1985. *CRC handbook of medicinal herbs.* Boca Raton, FL: CRC Press, Inc.

_____. 1987. *Handbook of Northeastern Indian medicinal plants.* Lincoln, Massachusetts: Quarterman Publications, Inc.

Eilmes, H.G. 1976. *Antivirale Wirkung von Pflanzeninhaltsstoffen am Beispiel von Echinacea angustifolia un Flavonoiden.* Dissertation, Frankfurt/Main.

Ellingwood, F. 1902. *A systematic treatise on materia medica and therapeutics.* Chicago: Chicago Medical Press Co.

_____. 1905. *Echinacea angustifolia. Therap. Gazette, Detroit* 21:298–300.

_____. 1914. Echinacea: The vegetable antitoxin, its characteristics, and peculiar therapeutic effects. *Am. Jour. Clin. Med.* 21(11):987–93.

_____. 1915. *American materia medica, therapeutics and pharmacognosy.* Chicago: Ellingwood's Therapeutist.

Enbergs, H. and A. Woestmann. 1986. *Tierärztl Umschau* 41:878–85.

Erpenbach, W. 1954. *Madaus Jahresbericht* 8:7–19.

Ewan, J., and N. Ewan. 1970. *John Banister and his natural history of Virginia 1678–1692.* Chicago: University of Illinois Press.

Farnsworth, N. R. and R. W. Morris 1976. Higher plants — the sleeping giant of drug development. *Amer. J. Pharm.* 148:46–52.

Farnsworth, N. R. and D. D. Soejarto. 1985. Potential consequence of plant extinction in the United States on the current and future availability of prescription drugs. *Economic Botany* 39(3):231–40.

Federal Register. 1979. Determination that *Echinacea tennesseensis* is an endangered species. 44(110): 32604–5 (June 6).

Felder, H. 1959. *Med. Klinik* 54:525–26.

Felter, H.W. 1898. The newer materia medica. I. Echinacea. *Eclectic Medical Journal* 58:79–89.

———. ed. 1901. *Syllabus of Eclectic materia medica and therapeutics.* Cincinnati: Scudder Brothers Company.

———. 1902. *History of the Eclectic Medical Institute, Cincinnati, Ohio — 1845–1902.* Cincinnati: The Alumnal Association of the Eclectic Medicial Institute.

Felter, H. W. and J. U. Lloyd. 1898. *King's American dispensatory.* 18th ed. Reprint ed. 1983. Portland, Oregon: Eclectic Medical Publications.

———. 1905. *King's American dispensatory.* 19th ed. Cincinnati: The Ohio Valley Co.

Felter, H.W. and J.T. Lloyd. (n.d). *Echinacea.* Cincinnati: Lloyd Brothers, Pharmacists, Inc.

Fernald, M.L. 1900. Notes on Echinacea. *Rhodora* 2:84–87.

———. 1950. *Gray's manual of botany.* 8th ed. New York: D. Van Nostrand.

Fischer. 1939. *Z. ärtzl. Fortbildung.* 36.

Fish, P.A. 1993. Echinacea in veterinary practice. *Am. Vet. Rev.* 27(8):716–26.

Flexner, A. 1910. *Medical education in the United States and Canada.* Carnegie Endowment Bulletin Number 4. New York: Carnegie Endowment.

Foster, S. 1984a. *Herbal bounty —the gentle art of herb culture.* Layton, Utah: Gibbs M. Smith, Inc.

———. 1984b. Flowering Panacea. *Harrowsmith* 55:124–25.

———. 1984c. *Echinacea Exalted! The botany, culture, history and medicinal uses of the purple coneflower.* Drury, Missouri: Ozark Beneficial Plant Project, New Life Farm, Inc.

———. 1984d. The Woods of Ozark County Abound in Beneficial Herbs. *Ozark County Times* (Wednesday, July 25):9.

———. 1985a. Herb Traders Beware. *Herbalgram* 2(1):3.

———. 1985b. Echinacea—An honest appraisal. *Business of Herbs* (March/April):8–10.

———. 1985c. Echinacea. *American Horticulturist* (August):14–17.

———. 1985d. *Echinacea exalted—the botany, culture, history, and medicinal uses of the purple coneflowers.* 2nd. ed. Brixey, Missouri: Ozark Beneficial Plant Project.

———. 1987a. Echinacea quality control monograph—a literature review. American Herbal Products Association Standards Committee.

———. 1987b. American herbs — our neglected heritage. In *Proceedings of the second national herb growing and marketing conference,* eds. J.E. Simon and L. Grant, pp. 265–72. West Lafayette, Indiana: Purdue Research Foundation.

_____. 1987c. Echinacea—what is the best species? *Am. Herb Assn. Newsletter* 5(2):4.

_____. 1988. The markets for native American plants: ideas and considerations. In *The Proceedings of the third national herb growing and marketing conference,* eds. A.K. Kestner and M.A. Buehrle, pp. 36: 1–11. Silver Springs, PA: IHGMA.

_____.1989a. Phytogeographic and botanical considerations of medicinal plants disjunct in Eastern Asia and Eastern North America. In *Herbs, spices, and medicinal plants: recent advances in botany, horticulture, and pharmacology.* Vol. 4, eds. L.E. Craker and J.E. Simon, pp. 115–40. Phoenix: Oryx Press.

_____. 1989b. Echinacea — more than just another pretty flower. *Bestways* (April):40–41.

_____. 1989c. Fact sheet on Echinacea species: *Echinacea angustifolia, Echinacea purpurea, Echinacea pallida.* Helena, Montana: Great Northern Botanicals Assn.

_____. 1990a. *Echinacea: the purple coneflowers.* American Botanical Council Botanical Series #301.

_____. 1990b. Echinacea in the herb garden. *The Herb Companion* (October/November):33–38.

Foster, S. and J.A. Duke.1990. *A field guide to medicinal plants: eastern and central North America.* Boston: Houghton Mifflin Co.

Franken, E. and N. Soennichsen. 1966. *Aesthet. Med.* 15:242–45.

Freyer, H. U. 1974. *Fortschr. Med.* 52:165–68.

Fyfe, J.W. 1909. *Specific diagnosis and specific medication.* Cincinnati: The Scudder Brothers Company.

Gaertner, W. 1968. *Landartz* 39(3):123–24.

Gaisbauer, M. and W. Zimmerman. 1986. *Natura Med.* 1:6–10.

Gaisbauer, M. Th. Schleich, H. Stickl, and W. Zimmerman. 1987. *Natura Med.* 1:6–12.

Gathercoal, E.N. and E. H. Wirth. 1949. *Pharmacognosy.* 2nd. ed. Philadelphia: Lea & Febiger.

Gattinger, A. 1894. *The medicinal plants of Tennessee.* Nashville: Tennessee Dept. of Agric.

Giesbert. 1943. *Fortschr. Ther.* 19:4.

Gilmore, M.R. 1909. Ethnobotany of the Omaha Indians. Unpublished master's thesis, University of Nebraska.

_____. 1913a. A study of the ethnobotany of the Omaha Indians. *Collections Neb. St. His. Soc.* 17:314–57.

_____. 1913b. Some native Nebraska plants with their uses by the Dakota. *Collections Neb. St. His. Soc.* 17:358–70.

_____. 1919. Uses of plants by Indians of the Missouri River region. In *33rd Annual Report of the Bureau of American Ethnology,* pp. 43–124.Washington, D.C.: Smithsonian Institution. [Reprinted 1977 University of Nebraska Press, Lincoln].

The Gleaner. 1928a. 32 (Feb.): 1050, 1053–54.

_____. 1928b. 33 (Aug.): 1079.

_____. 1931. 38 (April): 1204, 1210, 1222.

_____. 1934. 42 (Feb.): 1326–27.

Gleason, H.A. 1952. *The new Britton and Brown illustrated flora of the Northeastern United States and adjacent Canada.* 3 vols. New York: The New York Botanical Garden.

Gleason, H.A. and A. Cronquist. 1963. *Manual of the vascular plants of the Northeastern United States and adjacent Canada.* New York: Van Nostrand.

Goss, I.J.M. 1889. *A text book of materia medica, pharmacology, and special therapeutics.* Chicago: W.T. Keener.

Gray, A. 1848. *A manual of botany of the Northeastern United States.* Boston: James Munroe and Co.

_____. 1870. *School and field book of botany.* New York: Ivison, Blakeman, and Taylor.

_____. 1880. *Manual of botany of the Northeastern United States.* 5th ed. New York: Ivison, Blakeman, and Taylor.

Grieve, M. 1931. *A modern herbal.* 2 vols. Reprint ed. 1971. New York: Dover.

Griggs, B. 1982. *Green Pharmacy.* New York: Viking.

Grinnell, G.B. 1923. *The Cheyenne Indians: their history and ways of life.* 2 vols. New Haven: Yale University Press.

Gronovius, J.F. 1739. *Flora Virginica.* Part 1 Leiden: Cornelium Haak.

Gronovius, L.T. 1762. *Flora Virginica.* 2nd. ed. Reprint ed. 1946. Cambridge, MA: Arnold Arboretum.

Günther, E., E. F. Heeger, and C. Rosenthal. 1952. *Pharmazie* 7:24–50.

Haase, H. 1940. *Deutsch Zahnärztliche Wochenschrift* 43(50):1–15.

_____. 1943. *Deutsch Zahnärztliche Wochenschrift* 46:349.

Hahn, G. and A. Mayer. 1984. *Österreichische Apotheker-Zeitung* 38(51/52): 1040–46.

_____. n.d. *Med. Biol. Schrift.* 13:22–23.

Halstead, B. W. and L. L. Hood. 1984. Natural methods to enhance immunity. *Bulletin of the Oriental Healing Arts Institute* 9(8):371–411.

Hansen, P. 1965. *Prophylaxe* 4(233): 278–81.

Hare, Caspari, and Rusby. 1905. *The national standard dispensatory.* Philadelphia: Henry C. Lea and Sons.

Harnischfeger, G. and Stolze. 1980. *Notabene Medici. Verlag Phamamedolingua* 10:484.

Hart, J.A. 1976. Montana: native plants and early peoples. Helena: Montana Historical Society.

————. 1981. The ethnobotany of the northern Cheyenne Indians of Montana. *J. Ethnopharmacol.* 4:1–55.

Hartwell, J.L. 1969. Plants used against cancer. *Lloydia* (32):153–205.

Hartzell, A. 1947. Plant products for insecticidal properties and a summary of results to date. *Contri. Boyce Thompson Inst.* 15:21–34.

Hauberrisser, E. 1940. *Hippokrates* 11(17):393–398.

————. 1941. *Deutsche Zahnärztliche Wochenschrift* 44(11):153–58.

Hayden, F.V. 1859. Botany. In *Report of the Secretary of War,* 35th Congress, 2nd Session, 1858–1879, Senate Executive Document, Vol. 3, No. 1, Part 3, pp. 726–47.

Hayes, J.S. 1888a. *Echinacea angustifolia. Eclectic Medical Journal* Art. XVI: 68.

————. 1888b. *Echinacea angustifolia. Eclectic Medical Journal* (1888):142.

Heesen, W. 1964. *Erfahrungsheilk.* 13(5):210–17.

Heinzer, F., M. Chavanne, J.-P. Meusy, H.-P. Maitre, E. Giger, and T. W. Bauman. 1988. *Pharma. Acta. Helv.* 63:132–136.

Heizner, F., J.-P. Meusy, and M. Chavanne. 1989. *Echinacea pallida* and *Echinacea purpurea:* Follow-up of weight development and chemical composition for the first two culture years. *Planta Medica* 55:221.

Helbig, G. 1961. *Med. Klinik* 56:1512–14.

Heller. 1900. *Muhlenbergia* 1:5.

Hemmerly, T.E. 1976. Life cycle strategy of a highly endemic cedar glade species: *Echinacea tennesseensis* (Compositae). Ph.D. Dissertation. Vanderbilt University, Nashville, Tennessee.

————. 1986. Life cycle strategy of the highly endemic cedar glade species: *Echinacea tennesseensis. ASB Bulletin* 33(4):193–99.

Hemmerly, T.E. and E. Quarterman. 1978. Optimum conditions for the germination of seeds of cedar glade plants: a review. *Jour. Tenn. Acad. Sci.* 53(1):7–11.

Henkel, A. 1907. *American root drugs*. USDA, Bureau of Plant Industry, Bull. No. 107. Washington, D.C.: Government Printing Office.

Hepburn, *et. al.* 1950. Laboratory studies of twenty drugs on normal human beings, with comments on their symptomology and therapeutic use. *Jour. Am. Inst. Homeopathy*. 43:73–80.

Herrmann, G. 1952. *Münch. Med. Wschr.* 94(9):1–10.

Hertzel, H.N. 1944. *Deutsch. Med. Wochschr.* (701/2):6–9.

Hesse, M.C. 1973. Germination of seven species of wild flowers as affected by different pregermination conditions. Master's thesis. U. of Neb., Lincoln.

Heubl, G.R. and R. Bauer. 1989. *Deutsche Apotheker Zeitung* 129:2497–99.

Heubl, G.R, R. Bauer, and H. Wagner. 1988. *Sci. Pharm.* 56:145–60.

Heyl, F.W. and M.C. Hart. 1915. Some constituents of *Brauneria angustifolia. Jour. Am. Chem. Soc.* 37(7):1769–78.

Heyl, F.W. and J.F. Staley. 1914. Analyses of two Echinacea roots. *Am. Jour. Pharm.* 86:450–55.

Hind, N. 1987. *Echinacea purpurea. The Kew Magazine* 4(1):34–35.

Hipps, C. B. 1988. Purple coneflower: A dependable, late-summer-blooming native for the flower garden. *Horticulture* (August):46–49.

Hitchcock, C. L. and A. Cronquist. 1955. *Vascular plants of the Pacific Northwest* Vol. 5 (p. 160). Seattle: University of Washington Press.

———. 1981. *Flora of the Pacific Northwest*. Seattle: University of Washington Press.

Hocking, G.M. 1965. *Echinacea angustifolia* as a crude drug. *Quart. Jour. of Crude Drug Res.* 5(1):679–82.

Hobbs, C. 1989 *The Echinacea Handbook*. Portland, Oregon: Eclectic Medical Publications.

Homeopathic Pharmacopoeia Convention of the United States. 1981. *The Homeopathic Pharmacopoeia of the United States*. Boston: Otis Clapp & Son.

———. 1989. *Homeopathic Pharmacopoeia of the United States*. Revision Service, June, 1989.

Hooker, W.J. 1861. *Echinacea angustifolia. Curtis's Botanical Magazine* Tab. 5281.

Hundsdorfer, N.W. 1954. *Aerztliche Praxis* 6(8):1–4.

Hunter, C. 1984. *Wildflowers of Arkansas*. Little Rock: Ozark Society Foundation.

Jacobson, M. 1954. Occurrence of pungent insecticidal principle in coneflower roots. *Science* 120:1028–29.

_____. 1967. Structure of echinacein, the insecticidal component of American coneflowers. *J. Org. Chem.* 32(5):1646–47.

Jacobson, M., R.E. Redfern, and G.D. Mills.1975. Naturally occurring insect growth regulators. *Lloydia* 36(6):473–76.

Jelitto. K. 1989. Seed germination. *Bull. Am. Rock Gard. Soc.* 47(1):33–41.

JAQA. 1988. Clinical uses of Echinacea. 4 (2): 6–7.

Jung, F. 1951. *Therap. Gegenw.* 90(1):9–13.

Jurcic, K., D. Melchart, M. Holzmann, P. Martin, R. Bauer, A. Doenecke, and H. Wagner. 1989. *Zeitschrift für Phytotherapie* 10:67–70.

Kabelik, J. 1965. *Ziva* 13(1):4–5.

Kärcher K. H. 1971. *Mitteilung von 4:10,* an Fa. Schaper & Brümmer.

Keller, H. 1958. Patent Chemie Grünenthal DBP - 930674 K1.15.1. C.A. 53: 8550 (1959).

Keller, H.G. 1962. "An Anatomical Study of the Genus Echinacea." Unpubl. master's thesis, University of Kansas.

Kessler, K. 1987. Coneflower: new roles for an old plant? *The Furrow* 92(5):30.

Khan, I.A. 1987. *Neue sesquiterpenester aus Parthenium integrifolium L. und polyacetylene aus Echinacea pallida* Nutt. Unpubl. Ph.D. dissertation, University of Munich.

Kigour, J.C. 1897. Lobelia and Echinacea. *Eclectic Medical Journal* 57(11):595–98.

Kindscher, K. 1989. Ethnobotany of purple coneflower (*Echinacea angustifolia,* Asteraceae). *Economic Botany* 43(4):498–507.

King, J. and R.S. Newton. 1852. *The Eclectic dispensatory of the United States of America.* Cincinnati: H.W. Derby.

_____. 1887. Echinacea angustifolia. *Eclectic Medical Journal* 42:209–10.

Kinkel, H.J., M. Plate and U. Tüllner. 1984. *Med. Klinik* 79(21):580–83.

Kleinschmidt, H. 1965. *Therapie der Gegenwart* 104:1258–62.

Koch, E. 1940. *Hippokrates* 11:373–79.

Koch, E. and H. Haase. 1952. *Arzneimittel Forschung* 2:464–67.

Koch, E. and H. Uebel. 1953a. *Arzneimittel Forschung* 3:16–19.

_____. 1953b. *Arzneimittel Forschung* 3:133–37.

_____. 1954. *Arzneimittel Forschung* 4:551–60.

Korting, G.W. and W. Born. 1954. *Arzneimittel Forschung* 4:424–26.

Korting, G.W. and Rasp. 1954. *Medizinische* 45:1504–08.

Kraemer, H. 1912. Microscopy of Echinacea root. *Am. Druggist* (1912):23–24.

Kraemer, H. and M. Sollenberger. 1911. The pharmacognosy of Echinacea. *Am. Jour. Pharm.* 83:315–24.

Kral, R. 1983. *A report on some rare, threatened, or endangered forest-related vascular plants of the South.* 2 vols. Atlanta, GA: USDA, Forest Service.

Kriebisch. 1939. Dissertation. University of Cologne.

Krochmal, A., R.S. Walters and R.M. Doughty. 1971. *A guide to medicinal plants of Appalachia.* Agri. Handbook No. 400. Forest Service, USDA.

Kron, R. 1942. *Med. Klinik* 38(32):1315.

Kuhn, O. 1953. *Arzneimittel Forschung* 3:194–200.

Kühnast, R., E. Coeugniet, K. Schimmel, and A. Rodewald. 1986. *Ärzte Ztg.* 5(90):14.

Kunstmann, D.D. 1984. *Zeitschrift für Allgemeinmedizin* 60(11):528–29.

Lenk, W. 1989. *Zeitschrift für Phytotherapie* 10:49–51.

Liebstein, A.M. 1927. The therapeutic action of Echinacea. *Eclectic Medical Journal* 87:316–20.

Linnaeus, C.1753. *Species Plantarum.* vol. 2. reprint ed. 1959. The Ray Society, London.

Lindley, J. 1849. *Paxt Mag. Bot.* 15:79.

Little, G.W. 1917. An effective treatment for canine distemper. *Am. Journ. Vet. Med.* 12(10):691–94.

Lloyd, C.G. 1893. Should discoveries made by physicians be protected? *Annual of Eclectic Medicine and Surgery* 4:332–33.

———. 1897. Echinacea. *Eclectic Medical Journal* 424.

Lloyd, J.U. 1897. Empiricism Echinacea. *Eclectic Medical Journal* 57(8):421–27.

———. 1904a. History of *Echinacea angustifolia. Pharm. Rev.* 22(1):1–14.

———. 1904b. History of *Echinacea angustifolia. Am. Jour. Pharm.* 76(1):15–19.

———. 1912. Echinacea. *Jour. Am. Pharm. Assn.* 1:165.

———. 1921. Echinacea. *Am. Jour. Pharm.* 93:229.

———. 1924. *A treatise on Echinacea.* Drug Treatise No. 30. Cincinnati: Lloyd Brothers, Pharmacists, Inc.

Lloyd Brothers, Pharmicists, Inc. 1927. Facsimile reproductions of the principal labels of Specific Medicines. Cincinnati.

Löbe, J. and W. Schade. 1948. *Deutsches Gesundheitswesen* 4:117–18.

Lohmann-Matthes, M.-L. and H. Wagner. 1989. *Zeitschrift für Phytotherapie* 10:52–59.

Lorenz, E. and H. Messner. 1974. *Klin. Pädiat.* 186:37.

Lorenz, E., H. Messner, and I Mutz. 1972. Leucocytokinetic studies during viral hepatitis. *Zeitschrift F. Kinderheilkunde* 113(3):171–74.

Luettig, B, C. Steinmüller, G.E. Gifford, H. Wagner, and M.-L. Lohmann-Matthes 1989. Macrophage activation by the polysaccharide arabinogalactan isolated from plant cell cultures of *Echinacea purpurea. J. Natl. Cancer Inst.* 82(9): 669–75.

Lützenkirchen, A. 1952. *Die Medizinische* 27/28: 1–8.

Mabberly, D.J. 1981. *Taxon* 30(1):16.

Madaus, G. 1983. *Lehrbuch der biologischen Heilmittel.* 3 vols. Reprint ed. 1979. Liepzig: Georg Thieme Verlag.

Manidakis, G. 1968. *Echinacin-Test als Knochenmark-Funktionsprüfung vor und nach Strahlentherapie.* Dissertation. Heidelberg.

Mathews, A.B. 1905. Echinacea—some of its uses in modern surgery. *Gu. Pract.* 1(5):137–40.

May, G. and G. Willuhn. 1978. *Arzneimittel Forschung* 28:1–7.

McGregor, R.L. 1968a. The taxonomy of the genus Echinacea (Compositae). *Univ. of Kansas Science Bulletin* 48:113–42.

————. 1968b. A new species and two new varieties of Echinacea (Compositae). *Trans Kans. Acad. Sci.* 70:366–70.

————. 1968c. *Echinacea simulata. SIDA* 3:382.

Mears, J.A. 1975. The taxonomy of *Parthenium* section *Partheniastrum* DC. (Asteraceae-Ambrosiinae). *Phytologia* 31(6):463–82.

Medical Herbalism. 1990. News from Germany: contraindications for Echinacea? 2 (3): 6.

Meißner, F. K. 1980. *Medikamentöse Beeinflussung der Nekroserate von Hautluppen im Tierversuch.* Dissertation, Munich.

————. 1987. *Arzneimittel Forschung* 37(1):17–18.

Meißner, H.K.L. 1950a. *Medizin Heute* 11:1–3.

————. 1950b. *Ärtzl. Praxis.* 2:2.

————. 1951. *Die Therapiewoche* 9:522–23.

————. 1953. *Medizine Heute.* (1953):27.

Moell, O.H. 1951a. *Der Krankenhausartz* 8:1–4.

————. 1951b. *Therapiewoche Folge* 9:522.

Moench, C. 1794. *Methodas Planatas.* Marburgi Cattorum: In Officina Nova Libraria Academiae.

Moerman, D.E. 1977. *American Medical Ethnobotany.* New York: Garland Publishing Co.

————. 1981. *Geraniums for the Iroquois*. Algonac, MI: Reference Publications, Inc.

————. 1986. *Medicinal Plants of Native America*. 2 vols. Ann Arbor: University of Michigan Museum of Anthropology.

Moring, S.E. 1983. Echinacea—Natural remedy for viral infections. *Am. Herb. Assn. Quart. Newsletter* 2(2):5–6.

————. 1984. *Echinacea— a natural immune stimulant and treatment for viral infections*. Sunnyvale, CA: S.E. Moring.

Morison, R. 1699. *Plantarum historiae universalis oxoniensis*. Rt. 3, sec. 6, pl. 9.

Morton Arboretum. 1972. Notes on the propagation of plants (revised 7 February). Lisle, IL.

Möse, J.R. 1983. *Medwelt* 34 (51/52):1463–67.

Moser, Jr., J. 1910. Echinacea and a spurious root that appeared in the fall of 1909. *Am. Jour. Pharm.* 82:224.

Mostbeck, A. and M. Studlar. 1962. *Wiener Med. Wochenschrift.* 112(13):259–262.

Muennich, A. 1956. *Muench. Med. Wschr.* 98(15):528–31.

————. 1957/58. *Die Therapiewoche* 8(5).

Mund-Hoym, W.D. 1979. *Aerztl. Praxis* 31(14):566–67.

Munson, P.J. 1981. Contributions to Osage and Lakota ethnobotany. *Plains Anthropology* 26(3):229–40.

Necker, N.J. de. 1790. *Elementa Botanica*. 1:7.

Neugebauer, H. 1949. The constituents of Echinacea. *Pharmazie* 4:137–40.

Nicholson, G. 1885–1886. *The Illustrated Dictionary of Gardening*. Vol. 2. London: L. Upcott Gill.

Nickel, R.K. 1974. Plant resource utilization at a late prehistoric site in North central South Dakota. Unpubl. master's thesis, University of Nebraska, Lincoln.

Niederkorn, J.S. 1930. *A handy reference book*. Cincinnati: Lloyd Brothers Pharmacists, Inc.

Nikol'skaya, B.S. 1954. *Trudy Vsesoyuz. Obshchestva Fiziologov, Biokhimikov i Farmakologove Akad. Nauk. S.S.S.R.* 2:194–97.

Norton, J.B. 1902. Notes on some plants of the Southwestern United States *Trans. Acad. Sci. St. Louis* 7:40–41.

Nuttall, T. 1834. Descriptions of some of the rarer or little known plants indigenous to the United States, from dried specimens in the Herbarium of the Academy of Natural Sciences in Philadelphia. *Jour. Acad. Nat. Sci. Phil.* 7:77–80.

_____. 1841. Descriptions of new species and genera of plants in the natural order Compositae. *Trans. Am. Phil. soc. n. ser.* 7:354.

Orinda, D., J. Diederich, and A. Wacker. 1973. Antiviral activity of constituents of *Echinacea purpurea. Arzneimittel Forschung* 23(8):1119–20.

Orzechowski, G. 1962. *Der Deutche Apotheker* 14(9):1–12.

Ottoson, H.W. 1978. *Wildflowers for Nebraska landscapes.* The Agri. Exp. St., Univ. Neb., Lincoln.

Palmer, E. J. 1936. *Brauneria atrorubens* and *B. paradoxa. Rhodora* 38: 197–98.

Pappert, W. 1956. *Der Landarzt* 32(27): 666.

Philippart, R. 1944. *Korrespondenzblatt Für Zahnärtze* 5:7–14.

Plunkenett, L. 1696. *Opera omnia botanica IV. Almagestrum botanicum.* London.

Pohl, P. 1969. *Med. Klinik* 56:1546–47.

Proksch, A. 1980. *Über ein immunstimulierendes Wirkprinzip aus Echinacea purpurea. (L.)* Moench. Dissertation. University of Munich.

Proksch, A. and H. Wagner. 1987. Structural analysis of a 4-*O*-methyl-glucuronoarabinoxylan with immuno-stimulating activity from *Echinacea purpurea. Phytochemistry* 26(7):1989–93.

Quarterman, E. and T. E. Hemmerly. 1971. Rediscovery of *Echinacea tennesseensis* (Beadle) Small. *Rhodora* 73:304–5.

Quarterman, E. and P. Somers. 1984. The rare plants of middle Tennessee. *The Tennessee Conservationist* Vol. L. (2):11–13.

Radford, A. E., H.E. Ahles and C.R. Bell. 1968. *Manual of the vascular flora of the Carolinas.* Chapel Hill: Univ. of N.C. Press.

Rafinesque, C.S. 1825. *Neogenyton or indication of 66 new genera of plants of North America.* Lexington, KY: C.S. Rafinesque. 4 p.

_____. 1830. *Medical flora: manual of the medical botany of the United States of America.* Vol. 2. Philadelphia: Samuel C. Atkinson. [Listed on page 227 as "*Helichroa*"].

Range, W. 1969. *Medizin Heute* 18(4):111–13.

Reichart, M. 1983. *Psoralea esculenta* in Northeast Kansas. *Jour. Kansas Anthropological Assn.* 4(7&8):103–13.

Reith, F. J. 1978. Pharmaceuticals containing lactic acid derivatives and *Echinacea. Ger. Offen.* 10 pp.

Reuß, D. 1979. *Zschr. Allg. Med.* 55(24):1324.

————. 1981. *Zschr. Allg. Med.* 57(11):865.

————. 1986. *Rheuma.* 1986(5):29–32.

Riddle, J.L. 1834. A synopsis of the flora of the western states. *The Western Jour. of the Medical and Physical Sciences.*

Rigg, C.H. 1896. Echinacea. *Eclect. M.J. Cincinnati* lvi:166.

Robinson, B.L. and M.L. Fernald. 1908. *Gray's new manual of botany.* 7th ed. New York: American Book Company.

Roder, E., H. Wiedenfeld, Th. Hille, and R. Britz-Kirstgen. 1984. *Deutsche Apotheker Zeitung* 124:2316–18.

Röseler, W. 1952. *Die Medizinische* 3:1–10.

Rücker, G. 1963. *Pharm. Ztg.* 108:1169–75.

Ruland, A. 1942. *Deutche Zahnärztl. Wschr.* 45(40):535–40.

Salac, S., J.M. Traeger, and P.M. Jensen. 1982. Seeding dates and field establishment of wildflowers. *HortScience* 17(5):805–06.

Sartor, K.J. 1972. *Therapie der Gegenwart* 111:1147–50.

Sayre, L.E. 1897. Therapeutical notes and descriptions of parts of medicinal plants growing in Kansas. *Trans. Kans. Acad. Sci.* 16:85–89

————. 1898. Echinacea root. *Drugg. Circ.* 42:124–25.

————. 1903. Echinacea roots. *Trans. Kans. Acad. Sci.* 19:209–13.

————. 1904. Echinacea angustifolia. *Drugg. Circ.* 48:5.

————.1915. Cultivation of medicinal plants in the United States *Trans. Kans. Acad. Sci.* 27:110–13.

————. 1916. Cultivation of medicinal plants in the United States *Trans. Kans. Acad. Sci.* 28:133–36.

Schimmel, K., and G.T. Werner. 1981. *Therapie der Gegenwart* 120(11):1065–76.

Schimmer, O., G. Abel, and C. Behninger. 1989. *Zeitschrift für Phytotherapie* 10:39–42.

Schindler, H. 1940. *Pharm. Zentralh.* 81:589–94.

Schöpf, J.D. 1787. *Materia Medica Americana Potissimum Regni Vegetabilis.* Erlangen, Germany. Reprint. ed. 1903. Lloyd Library Bulletin No. 6, Reproduction Series No. 3, Cincinnati.

Schulte, K.E., G. Ruecher, and J. Perlick. 1967. *Arzneimittel Forschung* 17(7):825–29.

Schulthess, B., E. Giger, and T.W. Baumann. 1989. May achene analyses serve for species diagnosis in Echinacea? *Planta medica* 55:213.

Schnurbusch, F. 1955. *Z. Laryng. Rhinol. Otol.* 34:520.

Schuster, A. 1952. *Medizinische Monatsschrift* 7:453–55.

Seidel, K. and H. Kuobloch. 1957. Proof and comparison of the antiphlogistic effect of antirheumatic drugs. *Z. Rheumaforsch.* 16:231–38.

Sharp, W.M. 1935. A critical study of certain epappose genera of the Heliantheae-Vebesininae of the normal family Compositae. *Ann. Mo. Bot. Garden* 22:51–152.

Shemluck, M. 1982. Medicinal and other uses of the Compositae by Indians of the United States and Canada. *Jour. Ethnopharmacol.* 5:303–58.

Sherman, J.A. 1979. *The complete botanical prescriber.* Corvallis, OR: J.A. Sherman.

Sickel, K. 1971. *Ärtzl. Praxis* 23(5):201.

Siggelkow, H.A. 1942. *Hippokrates* 46:1176–79.

Simons, C.M. 1972. Lloyd Library. *Cincinnati Jour. Med.* 53:185–88.

Slawson, A. 1918. Serum of *Inula* and *Echinacea* in the treatment of canine distemper. *Jour. Am. Vet. Med. Assn.* 53(6):766–67.

Small, J.K. 1903. *Flora of the Southeastern United States.* 1st. ed. New York: J.K. Small.

Small, J.K. 1933. *Manual of the Southeastern Flora.* Chapel Hill: Univ. of N.C. Press.

Smith, E.B. 1978. *An Atlas and Annotated List of the Vascular Plants of Arkansas.* Fayetteville, AR: E. B. Smith.

Smith, H.H. 1928. Ethnobotany of the Meskwaki Indians. *Bulletin of the Public Museum of Milwaukee* 4(2):175–236.

Smith-Jochum, C.C. 1987. Germination requirements and field cultivation effects on the field establishment and oil extracts of three *Echinacea* species. Unpublished master's thesis. Kansas State University, Manhattan, Kansas.

Soicke, H., G. A. Hassen and K. Goerler. 1988. *Planta Medica* 1988(2):175–76.

Somers, P. 1983. Recovery plan for a cedar glade endemic, the Tennessee Coneflower, *Echinacea tennesseensis* (Asteraceae). *Natural Areas Journal* 3(4):56–58.

Sorensen, J.T. and D.J. Holden. 1974. Germination of prairie forb seed. *J. Range Mang.* 27:123–26.

Sprockhoff, O. 1964. *Landarzt* 40(27):1173–74.

Stafleu, F. A. 1971. *Linnaeus and the Linnaeans.* Utrecht: A. Oosthoek's Uitgeversmattschappij N.V.

Stawowczyck, A. and A. Karkozka. 1959. Some chemical properties of *Echinacea purpurea* and *E. pallida* and the alcoholatures from these plants. *Dissertationes Pharm.* 21:183–90.

Stephens, A.F. 1913. *The Gleaner* 1:113.

Steyermark, J.A. 1938. Two undescribed plants from Arkansas. *Rhodora* 40:71–72.

———. 1963. *Flora of Missouri.* Ames, IA: Iowa State Univ. Press.

Stimpel, M., A. Proksch, H. Wagner, and M.L. Lohman-Matthes. 1984. Macrophage activation and induction of macrophage cytotoxicity by purified polysaccharide fractions from *Echinacea purpurea. Infection and Immunity* 46(3):845–49.

Stockberger, W.W. 1935. *Drug plants under cultivation.* USDA Farmer's Bulletin No. 663. Washington, D.C.: Government Printing Office.

Stoll, A., J. Renz and A. Brack. 1950. Antibacterial substances II. Isolation and constitution of echinacoside, a glycoside from the roots of *Echinacea angustifolia. Helv. Chim. Acta.* 33:1877–93.

Stoll, A. and E. Seebeck. 1952. *Monit. Farm. Ter.* 58:1538.

Stuhr, E.T. 1933. *Manual of Pacific Coast drug plants.* Corvallis, Oregon: E.T. Stuhr.

Sussenguth, A. 1943. *Hippokrates* 14:51–52, 706–707.

Taber, C.W. 1970. *Taber's cyclopedic medical dictionary.* Philadelphia: F.A. Davis Company.

Tantaquidgeon, G. 1942. A study of Delaware Indian medical practices and folk beliefs. Pennsylvania Historical Commission.

Thomas, R. L. 1922. *The Eclectic practice of medicine.* Cincinnati: John K. Scudder.

Thorne, J.P. 1898. Echinacea (editorial) *Wisc. Med. Recorder* 1:231.

Thulcke. 1942. *Hippokrates* 13(22):419–23.

Tierra, M. 1980. *Way of Herbs.* New York: Simon and Schuster.

Toineeta, J. 1970. *Absarog-Issawau* (from the land of the Crows). Unpublished master's thesis. Montana State University, Bozeman, Montana.

Tragni, A. Tubaro, S. Melis and C.L. Galli. 1985. Evidence from two classic irritation tests for anti-inflammatory actions of a natural extract, Echinacina B. *Fd. Chem. Toxic.* 23(2):317–19.

Tronnier, H. 1967. *Münch. Med. Wschr.* 109: 2118.

Tubaro, A., E. Tragni, P. Del Negro, C.L. Galli and R. Della Loggia. 1986. Anti-inflammatory activity of a polysaccharide fraction of *Echinacea angustifolia. J. Pharm. Pharmacol.* 39:567–69.

Tucker, A. O., J. A. Duke and S. Foster. 1989. Botanical nomenclature of medicinal plants. In *Herbs, spices, and medicinal plants: recent advances in botany, horticulture, and pharmacology.* Vol. 4, eds. L.E. Craker and J.E. Simon, pp. 169–242. Phoenix: Oryx Press.

Tünnerhoff, F.K. and H.K. Schwabe. 1955–56. Animal and human studies on tissue changes after gelatin and thrombin implants. *Arzneimittel Forschung* 5: 201–4, 520–22 (1955); 6: 330–34 (1956).

Tyler, V. E. 1979. Plight of plant-drug research in the United States today. *Economic Botany* 33:377–83.

———. 1986. Plant drugs in the 21st century. *Economic Botany* 40:279–88.

———. 1987. *The new honest herbal* — a sensible guide to the use of herbs and related remedies. Philadelphia: George F. Sitckley Co.

———. 1989. The herbal regulatory dilemma: a proposed solution. Presented in Ottawa on October 12, 1989, as part of the Drugs Directorate Seminar Series, Health Protection Branch, Health and Welfare Canada.

Tyler, V. E., L. R. Brady, and J. E. Robbers. 1988. *Pharmacognosy* 9th ed. Philadelphia: Lea & Febiger.

Tyler V. E. and V. M. Tyler. 1987. John Uri Lloyd 1849–1936. *Journal of Natural Products* 50(1):1–8.

Tympner, K.D. 1978. *Münch. Med. Wschr.* 120(32/33):1055–56.

Unruh, V. von. 1915. *Echinacea angustifolia* and *Inula helenium* in the treatment of tuberculosis. *Nat. Eclec. Med. Assn. Quart.* (September):15.

USDA. 1952. *Manual for testing agricultural and vegetable seeds.* Agriculture Handbook No. 30. Washington, D.C.: Government Printing Office.

U.S. Fish and Wildlife Service. 1983. *Tennessee coneflower recovery plan.* Atlanta, GA: United States Fish and Wildlife Service.

———. 1989. Tennessee coneflower recovery plan. (revised 14 Nov., 1989). Asheville, NC: U.S. Fish and Wildlife Service.

Verelis, C. and H. Becker. 1977. N-Alkanes of *Echinacea angustifolia. Planta Medica* 31(3):288–89.

Vestal, P. and R.E. Schultes. 1939. *The economic botany of the Kiowa Indians.* Cambridge, MA: Botanical Museum, Harvard University.

Viehmann, P. 1978. *Erfahrungsheilkunde* 27(6): 353–58.

Voaden, D.J. and M. Jacobson. 1972. Tumor inhibitors 3. Identification and synthesis of an oncolytic hydrocarbon from American coneflower roots. *J. Med. Chem.* 15(6): 619–23.

Vogel, G. et. al. 1968. Evaluation of antiexudative Drugs. *Arzneimittel Forschung* 18(4):426–29.

Vogel, V. 1970. *American Indian medicine.* Norman: Univ. of Oklahoma Press.

Volz, G. 1957. *Therapie Der Gegenwart* 98(8).

Vömel, Th. 1985. *Arzneimittel Forschung* 35(2):1437–39.

Wacker, A. 1981. *Aerzteschrift F. Naturheilverfahren* 22(12):669–73.

Wacker, A. and A. Hilbig. 1978. *Planta Medica* 33(1):89–102.

Wagner, H. 1981. *Isolierung und chemische Struktur eines immunstimulierenden Wirkprinzips aus Echinacea.* Interdisciplinary Phytotherapie Symposium, Munich, April 1981.

————. 1984. Immunostimulants of fungi and higher plants. In *Natural Products and Drug Development,* Alfred Benzon Symposium 20, Compenhagan 1984, P. Krogsgaard-Larsen, S.B. Christensen, H. Kofod, eds. Compenhagan: Munksgaard.

————. 1986a. Examination of the immune-stimulation effect of some plant homeopathic drugs. *Biological Therapy* 4(2):21–27.

————. 1986b. *Natura Med.* 1:11–17.

Wagner, H. and A. Proksch. 1981a. An immunostimulating active principle from *Echinacea purpurea. A. Agnew. Phytother.* 2(5):166–68, 171.

————. 1981b. Isolation of polysaccharides with immunostimulating activity from *Echinacea purpurea. In Int. Conf. Chem. Biotechnil. Biol. Act. Nat. Prod. (Proc.),* B. Atanasove, ed. 3(1):2002.

————. 1985. Immunostimulatory drugs of fungi and higher plants. In *Economic and Medicinal Plant Research* Vol. 1., N. Farnsworth, H. Hikino and H. Wagner, eds., pp.113–155. Orlando, FL: Academic Press.

Wagner, H., A. Proksch, I. Riess-Maurer, A. Vollmar, S. Odenthal, H. Stuppner, K. Jurcic, M. Le Turdu and J.N. Fang. 1985. *Arzneimittel Forschung* 35(8):1069–75.

Wagner, H. *et. al.* 1982. Low molecular-weight polysaccharides from plants of the Composite family and pharmaceutical compositions contain them. *Germ. Offen.* DE 3,042,491.

Wagner, H., H. Stuppner, W. Schäfer and M. Zenk. 1988. Immunologically active polysaccharides of *Echinacea purpurea* cell cultures. *Phytochemistry* 27(1):119–26.

Wagner, H., H. Stuppner, J. Puhlmann, B. Brümmer, K. Deppe, and M.H. Zenk. 1989. *Zeitschrift für Phytotherapie* 10:35–38.

Wallace, G. 1987. Coneflower digging on state land. Missouri Department of Conservation Memorandum.

Watkins, L. 1895. *An Eclectic compendium of the practice of medicine.* Cincinnati: John M. Scudder's Sons.

Watson, S. and J.M. Coulter. 1889. *Gray's manual of botany.* 6th ed. New York: American Book Company.

Weaver, J. E. and T.J. Fitzpatrick. 1934. The Prairie. *Ecological Monographs* 4(2):214–15.

Webster, H.T. 1898. *Dynamical therapeutics.* San Francisco: Webster Medical Publishing Co.

Wedel, W.T. 1936. *An introduction to Pawnee archeology.* Smithsonian Institution, Bureau of American Ethnology, Bulletin 112. Washington, D.C.: Government Printing Office.

Weiss, F.R. 1988. *Herbal Medicine.* Translated by A.R. Meuss. Portland, Oregon: Medicina Biologica.

Weissbach, L. G. Wegner, and H. Schweikert. 1977. *Therapiewoche* 27:6009–21.

Wember, S. 1953. *Landarzt* 29: 621.

Woods, E.L. 1930. The chemical constitution of the hydrocarbons of *Echinacea angustifolia. Am. J. Pharm.* 102:611–30.

Zimmerman, O. 1969. *Hippokrates* 40(6):233–35.

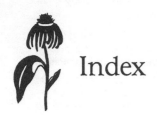

Index